The Evidence^{TM}

Revised Edition

Edited by
Jonathan Soverow, MD, MPH
Robert McGarrah, MD

Co-editors
Kathleen Finn, MD
Doug Wright, MD, PhD
Alberto Puig, MD, PhD

Dedicated to
the MGH
Housestaff and
their families

Contributing faculty

Daniel P. Hunt, MD, FACP
Chief, Hospital Medicine Unit, Massachusetts General Hospital
Director, Inpatient Clinician Educator Service, Department of Medicine, Massachusetts General Hospital
Associate Professor of Medicine, Harvard Medical School

William Kormos, MD
Education Director, John D. Stoeckle Center for Primary Care Innovation, Massachusetts General Hospital
Instructor in Medicine, Harvard Medical School

E. Kevin Heist, MD, PhD, MMSc
Cardiac Arrhythmia Service, Division of Cardiology, Department of Medicine, Massachusetts General Hospital
Assistant Professor of Medicine, Harvard Medical School

Sanjeev Francis, MD
Division of Cardiology, Department of Medicine, Massachusetts General Hospital
Instructor in Medicine, Harvard Medical School

James Januzzi, MD
Division of Cardiology, Department of Medicine, Massachusetts General Hospital
Director, Cardiac Intensive Care Unit
Associate Professor of Medicine, Harvard Medical School

Gregory D. Lewis, MD
Division of Cardiology, Department of Medicine, Massachusetts General Hospital
Associate Director, MGH Cardiopulmonary Exercise Laboratory, Massachusetts General Hospital
Assistant Professor of Medicine, Harvard Medical School

Jatin M. Vyas, MD, PhD
Division of Infectious Diseases, Department of Medicine, Massachusetts General Hospital
Assistant Professor of Medicine, Harvard Medical School

Mark C. Fisher, MD, MPH
Division of Rheumatology, Allergy and Immunology, Department of Medicine, Massachusetts General Hospital
Instructor in Medicine, Harvard Medical School

Edwin Choy, MD, PhD
Division of Hematology & Oncology, Department of Medicine, Massachusetts General Hospital
Director of Sarcoma Research, Division of Hematology & Oncology, Massachusetts General Hospital
Assistant Professor of Medicine, Harvard Medical School

Ednan Bajwa, MD, MPH
Division of Pulmonary & Critical Care, Department of Medicine, Massachusetts General Hospital
Associate Director, Medical Intensive Care Unit, Massachusetts General Hospital
Assistant Professor of Medicine, Harvard Medical School

Deborah Wexler, MD
Division of Endocrinology, Department of Medicine, Massachusetts General Hospital
Assistant Professor of Medicine, Harvard Medical School

Raymond Chung, MD
Division of Gastroenterology, Department of Medicine, Massachusetts General Hospital
Vice Chief, Gastroenterology Division, Massachusetts General Hospital
Director of Hepatology, Massachusetts General Hospital
Medical Director, Liver Transplant Program, Massachusetts General Hospital
Associate Professor of Medicine, Harvard Medical School

Senior Resident Section Editors

Neil Ahluwalia, MD

David Ain, MD

Aarti Asnani, MD

Lindsay Jubelt, MD

Ryan Kaple, MD

Gina Kruse, MD

Wilson Kwong, MD, MS

Eli Miloslavsky, MD

Sydney Montesi, MD

Vilas Patwardhan, MD

Krishna Reddy, MD

Cindy Ta, MD

Aaron Tande, MD

Glossary of terms

ACR	American College of Rheumatology
ACEi	Angiotensin Converting Enzyme Inhibitor
AF	Atrial Fibrillation
AKI	Acute Kidney Injury
ARB	Angiotensin Receptor Blocker
ARR	Absolute Risk Reduction
ASA	Aspirin
ATN	Acute Tubular Necrosis
AV	Atrio-Ventricular
BB	Beta-blocker
CHF	Congestive Heart Failure
CK	Creatinine Kinase
Cr	Creatinine
CV	Cardiovascular
CVVH	Continuous Veno-venous Hemofiltration
DM	Diabetes Mellitus
Dx	Diagnosis
d	Days
ESR	Erythrocyte Sedimentation Rate
ESRD	End Stage Renal Disease
GI	Gastrointestinal
GFR	Glomular Filtration Rate
HD	Hemodialysis
ICU	Intensive Care Unit
LBBB	Left Bundle Branch Block
mg	Milligrams
MI	Myocardial Infarction
mm	Millimeters
mos	Months
NSAIDS	Non-Steroidal Anti-Inflammatory Drugs
NNT/NNH	Number Needed to Treat/ Harm
po	Per os
PPM	Permanent Pacemaker
QD	Every day
QOD	Every other day
RA	Rheumatoid Arthritis
RCT	Randomized Controlled Trial
RR	Relative Risk
RRR	Relative Risk Reduction
SLE	Systemic Lupus Erythematosis
TIA	Transient Ischemic Attack
VF	Ventricular Fibrillation
yo	Years old
yr	Year

Introduction

"I am not accustomed to saying anything with certainty after only one or two observations"
--Andreas Vesalius (1514-1564)

In the 16th century, Vesalius revolutionized medical thought by overthrowing traditional faiths about the human body and focusing on his own painstaking dissections. His principles of skepticism and direct observation still hold true. And though our methods have improved, their results still merit the critical review he espoused. The promise of "evidence-based medicine"—that it roots clinical decision-making in the scientific method—is also its shortcoming. Due to economic, ethical, and other technical constraints, the scientific method cannot be applied to every individual or situation. When it is applied to people, it requires creative patient selection, study design, and statistical analysis to make an experiment internally valid.

So in the era of evidence-based medicine, the details behind the evidence matter. They define the validity and applicability of treatments and diagnostic tests, yet are often misconstrued and stretched to meet our patients' needs. Exploring the fine points of modern medicine's seminal clinical research, *The Evidence* tries to identify the limitations of applying particular studies to the sick individuals before us.

This book does not present clinical practice recommendations by its authors or the   . Massachusetts General Hospital. On the contrary, *The Evidence* aims to critically review the major clinical studies that influence how we treat patients.

Using the Consolidated Standards of Reporting Trials (CONSORT) checklist, each one-page summary in this book reduces its respective study to its essential components, interpreting them through a commentary section at the end. The summaries were drafted by medical residents at the Massachusetts General Hospital, reviewed by senior resident section editors and subspecialty faculty members, and then reviewed a final time by the chief editors and three faculty members in the Clinician Educator department. We structured the summaries using the CONSORT checklist because of its ease-of-use and because it has become an industry standard, refined by expert panels starting in 1993 and endorsed by over 600 medical journals worldwide. The commentary section analyzes each trial, placing it into context of other relevant research.

Though this book does not contain every article an internal medicine resident should know, it comprises what our authors and editors consider an essential core while including often-quoted studies with serious flaws. Selecting the most important articles of our time poses a tremendous challenge. Opinions differ widely, and new data, sometimes conflicting, enter the literature every day. Using a quantitative process, such as the number of times an article has been cited, often yields controversial studies and misses landmark trials that have become so definitive (rightly or wrongly) that they are no longer questioned, referenced, or repeated. We chose these articles through an iterative process. The chief editors made initial suggestions based upon citations from our housestaff manual; these titles were further refined by section editors and faculty. We aim to produce multiple editions throughout the years as more research becomes available and would appreciate any feedback you have on studies to include or remove from future versions. The book was originally conceived in 2010 and written and printed in 2011 at the Massachusetts General Hospital, where it underwent circulation and review over the following year. This publication represents a revised edition based on that review.

We would like to acknowledge the incredible work of our co-residents and contributing faculty. We have learned a lot by putting it together and hope you will, too. If nothing else, you should be surprised by what you read and want to look beneath the skin—as Vesalius did—of the dogma of our time.

Jonathan Soverow, MD, MPH
Senior Resident in Internal Medicine
Massachusetts General Hospital
Email: evidence.editor@gmail.com

CONTENTS

I. General Medicine

Symptom-triggered Treatment of Alcohol Withdrawal (JAMA 1994; 272:519) **1**
John Korman
Revised Cardiac Risk Index (Circulation 1999; 100:1043) **2**
Mary Zhang
Hormone Replacement Therapy: Women's Health Initiative (JAMA 2002; 288:321) **3**
Jonathan Soverow
Aspirin Primary Prevention: Physician's Health Study (NEJM 1989; 321:129) **4**
Robert McGarrah
Hypertension: ALLHAT (JAMA 2002; 288:2981) **5**
Gina Kruse
Cervical Cancer and the HPV Vaccine (NEJM 2002; 347:1645) **6**
Andrew Courtwright

Health Policy:
Regional Variations in Medicare Spending. Part 1 (Ann Int Med 2003; 138:273) **7**
Maria Han
Regional Variations in Medicare Spending. Part 2 (Ann Int Med 2003; 138:288) **8**
Maria Han
RAND Health Insurance Experiment (NEJM 1983; 309:1426) **9**
Andrew Courtwright
Breast Cancer Screening (Cancer 2006; 106:732) **10**
Lindsay Jubelt

II. Cardiology

Acute Coronary Syndromes (ACS):
Plavix in ACS: CURE (NEJM 2001; 345:494) **11**
Shweta Motiwala
Statins and ACS: PROVE IT-TIMI 22 (NEJM 2004; 350:1495) **12**
Mary Zhang
Aspirin and Heparin in ACS (NEJM 1988; 319:1105) **13**
Ralph DeBiasi
Beta-blocker in ACS: COMMIT (Lancet 2005; 366:1622) **14**
Deepa Kumaraiah
Medical Therapy vs. Stenting in Stable Angina: COURAGE (NEJM 2007; 356:1503) **15**
Deepa Kumaraiah

Arrhythmias:
Rate vs. Rhythm Control of Atrial Fibrillation: AFFIRM (NEJM 2002; 347:1825)   **16**
Jonathan Soverow
Amiodarone vs. Implantable Defibrillator for Heart Failure: SCD-HeFT   **17**
(NEJM 2005; 352:225)
Fernando Contreras
Implantable Defibrillator for Heart Failure: MADIT II (NEJM 2002; 346:877)   **18**
Fernando Contreras
Implantable Defibrillator after ACS: DINAMIT (NEJM 2004; 351:2481)   **19**
Aarti Asnani

Heart Failure:
Cardiac Resynchronization Therapy in Heart Failure: CARE-HF (NEJM 2005; 352:1539) **20**
Lauren Gilstrap
Spironolactone in Heart Failure: RALES (NEJM 1999; 341:709)   **21**
Lauren Gilstrap
Carvedilol vs. Metoprolol in Heart Failure: COMET (Lancet 2003; 362:7)   **22**
Shweta Motiwala

Prevention:
Statin Therapy for Secondary Prevention: 4S Study (Lancet 1994; 344:1383)   **23**
Aarti Asnani
C-Reactive Protein-Guided Statin Therapy: JUPITER (NEJM 2008; 359:2195)   **24**
Ralph DeBiasi

III. Infectious Diseases

Interrupted Antiretroviral Therapy: SMART (NEJM 2006; 355:2283)   **25**
Kemmy Mokoya
Early Antiretroviral Therapy: NA-ACCORD (NEJM 2009; 360:1815)   **26**
Rachel Bender
Antiretroviral Therapy with Tuberculosis: SAPIT (NEJM 2010; 362:697)   **27**
Emily Kendall
Steroids for Pneumocystis Pneumonia (NEJM 1990; 323:1451)   **28**
Allen Chang
Treatment of Ventilator-Associated Pneumonia (JAMA 2003; 290:2588)   **29**
Renee Rutledge
Steroids for *S. pneumoniae* Meningitis (NEJM 2002; 347:1549)   **30**
Sarah Turbett
Trans-Esophageal Echocardiogram for Endocarditis (JACC 1997; 30:1072)   **31**
Sarah Turbett
Pneumococcal Polysaccharide Vaccine (NEJM 2003; 348:1747)   **32**
Vernon Rayford
Treatment of Severe *C. difficile* Infection (CID 2007; 45:302)   **33**
David Lyckowski

French study Rx duration HCAP - 8d v 14d for Abx
└ No diff. except pseudomonas, acinetobacter (+stenotrophomonas)

IV. Rheumatology

Autoantibodies Before Onset of Systemic Lupus Erythematosis (NEJM 2003; 349:1526)   **34**
Laura Certain
Treatment Strategies for Rheumatoid Arthritis: the BeSt study   **35**
(Arthritis Rheum 2005; 52:3381)
Zach Wallace
Temporal Arteritis: Predictive Features (JAMA. 2002; 287:92)   **36**
Eli Miloslavsky
Infliximab in Rheumatoid Arthritis (Lancet 1999; 354:1932)   **37**
John Korman
Intraarticular steroids in Osteoarthritis (Arthritis Rheum 2003; 48:370)   **38**
Annie Lee
NSAIDS in Osteoarthritis (NEJM 1991; 325:87)   **39**
Annie Lee
Systemic Lupus Erythematosis Criteria (Arthritis Rheum 1982; 25:1271)   **40**
Zach Wallace

V. Hematology & Oncology

Hematology:
Transfusion Requirements in Critical Care: TRICC (NEJM 1999; 340:409)   **41**
Jonathan Peled
LMWH vs. Warfarin for Venous Thromboembolism in Cancer: CLOT   **42**
(NEJM 2003; 349:146)
David Sallman
Clinical Factors and Recurrent Venous Thrombotic Events (JAMA 2005; 293:2352)   **43**
Andrew Brunner
Plasma Exchange Thrombotic Thrombocytopenic Purpura (NEJM 1991; 325:393)   **44**
Jonathan Soverow
Dexamethasone for Idiopathic Thrombocytopenic Purpura (NEJM 2003; 349:831)   **45**
Daria Babushok
Oncology:
All-*trans* Retinoic Acid in Acute Promyelocytic Leukemia (NEJM 1997; 337:1021)   **46**
Andrew Brunner
BCR-ABL Tyrosine Kinase Inhibitor in Chronic Myeloid Leukemia   **47**
(NEJM 2001; 344:1031)
Sheheryar Kabraji
EGFR Receptor Mutations Underlying Responsiveness of Lung Cancer Therapy   **48**
(NEJM 2004; 350:2129)
Aparna Mani
Early Palliative Care for Lung Cancer (NEJM 2010; 363:733)   **49**
Areej El-Jawahri
Mutations and Treatment Outcome in Cytogenetically Normal Acute Myeloid Leukemia   **50**
(NEJM 2008; 358:1909)
Paul Krezanoski

Temporary Remissions in Acute Leukemia (NEJM 1948; 238:787)   51
Tara Albano

VI. Nephrology

Darbepoetin in Chronic Kidney Disease (NEJM 2009; 361:2019)   52
Meghan Sise
Octreotide/midodrine in Hepatorenal Syndrome (Hepatology 1999; 29:1690)   53
Meghan Sise
ACEi/ARB Combination Treatment in Chronic Kidney Disease: ONTARGET   54
(Lancet 2008; 372:547)
Andrew Allegretti
ACEi vs. ARB Treatment Treatment in Diabetes and Chronic Kidney Disease   55
(NEJM 2004; 351:1952)
Opeyemi Olabisi
Early vs. Late Initiation of Hemodialysis (NEJM 2010; 363:609)   56
Opeyemi Olabisi
Intensity of Renal Support in Critically Ill (NEJM 2008; 359:7)   57
Andrew Allegretti

VII. Pulmonary & Critical Care

Pulmonary:
 Salmeterol and Fluticasone propionate in Chronic Obstructive Pulmonary Disease: 58
TORCH (NEJM 2007; 356:775)
Susan Mathai
Systemic Glucocorticoids and Chronic Obstructive Pulmonary Disease: SCCOPE   59
(NEJM 1999; 340:1941)
Mihir Parikh
Non-invasive Ventilation for Acute Chronic Obstructive Pulmonary Disease   60
(Lancet 2000; 355:1931)
Marjory Bravard
Inferior Vena Cava Filters and Pulmonary Embolism: PREPIC   61
(Circulation 2005; 112:416)
Mihir Parikh
Alteplase in Submassive Pulmonary Embolism (NEJM 2002; 347:1143)   62
Susan Mathai

Critical Care:
Low Tidal Volume Ventilation in Acute Respiratory Distress Syndrome   63
(NEJM 2000; 342:1301)
Ian Barbash
Fluid-management Strategies in Acute Respiratory Distress Syndrome: FACTT   64
(NEJM 2006; 354:2564)
Jessica Volk
Neuromuscular Blockers in ARDS (NEJM 2010; 363: 1107)   65
Katie Famous

Early Goal-directed Therapy in Septic Shock (NEJM 2001; 345:1368)   66
Katie Famous
Hydrocortisone Therapy in Septic Shock: CORTICUS (NEJM 2008; 358:111)   67
Robert McGarrah
Albumin vs. Saline for Fluid Resuscitation in the ICU: SAFE (NEJM 2004; 350:2247)   68
Marjory Bravard
Intensive Glucose Control in the ICU: NICE-SUGAR (NEJM 2009; 360:1283)   69
Susan Mathai
Sedation Status in the ICU (JAMA 2003; 289:2983)   70
Laura Brenner
Daily Interruption of Sedation in Mechanical Ventilation (NEJM 2000; 342:1471)   71
Neil Ahluwalia
Awakening and Breathing Controlled Trial for Ventilator Weaning: ABC   72
(Lancet 2008; 371: 126)
Krishna Reddy

VIII. Endocrinology

Calcium and Vitamin D: Women's Health Initiative (NEJM 2006; 354:669)   73
Cindy Ta
Avandia and Cardiovascular Risk (NEJM 2007; 356:2457)   74
James Young
Intensive Glucose Control in Type 2 Diabetes Mellitus: DCCT (NEJM 1993; 329:977)   75
Kelly Lauter
Intensive Glucose Control in Type 2 Diabetes Mellitus: UKPDS (Lancet 1998; 352:837)   76
Susan Mathai
Basal-bolus Insulin in Inpatient Diabetes Mellitus Management: RABBIT-2   77
(Diabetes Care 2007; 30:2181)
Taison Bell
Effects of Intensive Glucose-lowering in Type 2 Diabetes Mellitus: ACCORD   78
(NEJM 2008; 358:2545)
Dina Reiss
Zoledronic Acid for Osteoporosis: HORIZON Pivotal Fracture Trial   79
(NEJM 2007; 356:1809)
Marc Wein

IX. Gastroenterology

Intravenous Proton Pump Inhibitor in Gastrointestinal Bleeding (NEJM 2007; 356:1631) **80**
Amit Desai
Octreotide and Variceal Bleeding (Lancet 1995; 346:1666) **81**
John Holden
Steroids in Alcoholic Hepatitis (NEJM 1992; 326:507) **82**
Tian Gao
N-Acetylcysteine for Non-Acetaminophen Acute Liver Failure (Gastro 2009; 137:856) **83**
Jessica Ravikoff
Albumin and Spontaneous Bacterial Peritonitis (NEJM 1999; 341:403) **84**
Jonathan Soverow
Rifaximin for Hepatic Encephalopathy (NEJM 2010; 362:1071) **85**
Zachory Zator
Norfloxacin for Infection Prophylaxis with in Gastrointestinal Bleeding and **86**
Cirrhosis (Gastro 1992; 103:1267)
Michelle Long

INDIVIDUALIZED TREATMENT FOR ALCOHOL WITHDRAWAL: A RANDOMIZED DOUBLE-BLIND
CONTROLLED TRIAL
Saitz R, Mayo-Smith M, Roberts M, et al.
Journal of the American Medical Association. 1994; 272: 519

Summary: Symptom-triggered is superior to fix-scheduled chlordiazepoxide dosing for management of ethanol withdrawal.

Introduction: Fix-scheduled (FS) dosing of benzodiazepines for treatment of alcohol withdrawal may excessively sedate and prolong hospital stay.

Objective: "To assess the effect of an individualized treatment regimen on the intensity and duration of medication treatment for alcohol withdrawal."

Methods
Trial Design: Randomized, single-center (New Hampshire)
Participants: Veterans with a history of alcohol abuse/dependence admitted for withdrawal. Excluded: acute medical or psychiatric disease; seizure history; inability to take PO meds; unable/unwilling to consent; use/withdrawal from opiates, benzodiazepines, barbiturates, clonidine, or beta blockers
Interventions: FS group: chlordiazepoxide (CDE) 50mg x4 doses, then 25mg x 8 with 25-100mg q1hr PRN CIWA-Ar$\geq$8 (Clinical Institute Withdrawal Assessment for Alcohol scale, revised) vs. Symptom-triggered (ST) group: CDE 25-100mg Q1H PRN CIWA-Ar$\geq$8
Outcomes: Primary: duration and total dose of CDE treatment; Secondary: number/amount of as needed benzodiazepine doses; severity of alcohol withdrawal; leaving hospital against medical advice (AMA); development of seizures, hallucinations or delirium tremens (DTs); lethargy; discomfort and craving for alcohol; rates of rehabilitation, readmission and compliance with follow-up
Sample size: 101; 90% power to detect 12-hr decrease in duration of therapy

Randomization: Blocks of 10 patients randomly assigned to treatment group
Blinding: Double-blinded
Statistical methods: Intention-to-treat analysis; Kaplan-Meier curve; log rank, Wilcoxon test, student's *t* test, Fisher's Exact test

Results
Participant flow: 111 patients randomized; 5 left AMA (3 in FS group)
Baseline data: No significant differences
Outcomes and estimation: Median duration of CDE therapy and total CDE both less in ST vs. FS groups (9 vs. 68 hours, p<0.001; 100mg vs. 425mg, p<0.001, respectively). No differences were observed between the two groups for the prespecified secondary outcomes.
Harms: Respiratory depression in 1 FS patient

Discussion
Conclusion: ST therapy is equally effective but leads to decreased CDE use and duration of hospital stay compared to FS CDE taper
Limitations: Not powered to detect differences in outcomes (DTs, seizures, etc.); study took place in specialized hospital detoxification unit; nearly all male sample; numerous exclusions (seizures, acute medical/psych problems, etc.)

Funding: Roche Laboratories, Nutley, NJ [manufacturers of Librium (chlordiazepoxide)]

<u>Commentary</u>   *John Korman, MD, Resident in Internal Medicine*
This study confirms the importance of an individualized rather than one-size-fits-all approach to alcohol withdrawal. Benzodiazepine titration should be symptom-focused (in this case, using a modified CIWA-Ar score, incorporating sweating, agitation, anxiety, disorientation, nausea/vomiting, auditory/tactile/visual disturbances, tremor, and headache) with careful avoidance of over-sedation and its resultant risks. The study's primary limitation is the exclusion of patients with any active medical or psychiatric issues, seizure history, and co-substance withdrawal, which comprise a substantial portion of withdrawal patients admitted to the hospital. Likewise, subject homogeneity (middle-aged, male veterans) and absent quantification of daily alcohol consumption or serum ethanol levels are notable. These aspects impair generalizability but do not detract from the importance of symptom-focused management and its impact on treatment efficacy, patient safety, and health system savings.

DERIVATION AND PROSPECTIVE VALIDATION OF A SINGLE INDEX FOR PREDICTION OF CARDIAC RISK OF
MAJOR NONCARDIAC SURGERY (RCRI)
Lee TH, Marcantonio ER, Mangione CM, et al.
Circulation. 1999; 100: 1043

Summary: The 6 preoperative risk predictors identified by the Revised Cardiac Risk Index (RCRI) are: high-risk surgery (intraperitoneal, intrathoracic, suprainguinal vascular), history of CHF, stroke, ischemic heart disease, insulin-treated diabetes mellitus, and creatinine > 2.0mg/dL. Risk of major cardiac event increased with each predictor from 0.5% with 0 predictors to 11% with 3 or more predictors.

Introduction Cardiovascular complications cause significant morbidity following non-cardiac surgeries. The risk stratification tools available at the time of this study were complex and derived from small cohorts.

Objective: "To derive and validate a simple index for the prediction of the risk of cardiac complications in major elective noncardiac surgery."

Methods

Trial Design: Single-center study; retrospective derivation and prospective validation cohort
Participants: Adults ≥age 50 undergoing nonurgent, noncardiac surgery at a large academic teaching hospital (1989-1994) with an expected stay ≥2 days
Outcomes: Major cardiac complications: MI (by CK-MB criteria), pulmonary edema (CXR), ventricular fibrillation, or primary cardiac arrest, and complete heart block
Sample size: 2/3 (N=2893) in derivation cohort; 1/3 (N=1422) for prospective validation
Statistical methods: Univariate comparisons identified associations between clinical characteristics and outcomes. Logistic regression was used to create a set of independent correlates for the index. An index with variable weights assigned to the clinical correlates and an index with equal weights were compared using receiver operating characteristic curves (ROC).

Results
Baseline data: Similar between cohorts
Outcomes: The 6 predictors of cardiac complications had statistically significant odds ratios for cardiac complications in both the derivation and validation set, with the exception of insulin therapy and serum Cr levels.

**% risk of major cardiac complications
(Derivation-Validation)**

0 risk factor	0.4-0.5%
1 risk factor	0.9-1.3%
2 risk factors	3.6-6.6%
≥3 risk factors	9.1-11.0%

There was no significant difference in performance using ROC curves when indexes used variably weighted or equally weighted risk factors.

Discussion
Conclusion: In patients undergoing major, non-urgent, non-cardiac surgery, having ≥2 risk factors prospectively identified patients at moderate (7%) and high (11%) risk of cardiac complication.
Limitations: Several risk factors (advanced age, critical aortic stenosis, and arrhythmias) identified in previous studies did not correlate with complications. Not applicable to low risk procedures or emergency operations and limited statistical power for AAA surgeries (N=110). Limited generalizability given single center study with validation cohort from the same patient population
Funding: Agency for Health Care Policy and Research

Commentary *Mary H. Zhang, MD, Resident in Internal Medicine*
This study derived and validated the six elements of the Revised Cardiac Risk Index, demonstrating that it could be used prospectively to predict the likelihood of adverse cardiac events in patients undergoing noncardiac surgery. Later studies (a retrospective study by Lindenauer *et al* in 660,000 adults in *CMAJ* 2005;173:627 and the randomized POISE trial in *Lancet* 2008;371:1839) revealed higher event and mortality rates at the same RCRI risk level than predicted in this original paper. These differences may be attributable to the inclusion of sicker patients and emergent surgeries, as well as the use of the more sensitive troponin assay rather than CK-MB to diagnose MI. ACC/AHA guidelines for perioperative assessment incorporate the RCRI in preoperative evaluation, but the index may not apply to emergent surgeries and very old patients, which were not represented in validation studies. A newer risk calculator that includes age has been studied and may have improved performance characteristics compared with the RCRI [*Circulation* 2011; 124:381].

RISKS AND BENEFITS OF ESTROGEN PLUS PROGESTIN IN HEALTHY POSTMENOPAUSAL WOMEN:
PRINCIPAL RESULTS FROM THE WOMEN'S HEALTH INITIATIVE RANDOMIZED CONTROLLED TRIAL
Writing group for the Women's Health Initiative
Journal of the American Medical Association. 2002; 288: 321

Summary: In postmenopausal women, the overall risks of estrogen/progestin for primary prevention surpass the benefits over 5 years of follow-up.

Introduction
Observational studies suggest that combined hormone replacement therapy (HRT) may reduce coronary heart disease (CHD), but no randomized controlled trial had quantified its risks.

Objective: "To assess the major health benefits and risks of the most commonly used combined hormone preparation in the United States"

Methods
Trial Design: Randomized, multicenter (40 centers in US)
Participants: Healthy postmenopausal women aged 50-79 with intact uterus
Interventions: Estrogen (0.625mg/d) + medroxyprogesterone (2.5mg/d) vs. placebo
Outcomes: Nonfatal myocardial infarction and CHD death (primary); invasive breast cancer (primary adverse outcome); index of the 2 primary outcomes, stroke, pulmonary embolism, endometrial or colorectal cancer, hip fracture, and death
Sample size: 16,608; power calculations not provided
Randomization: Block randomization, stratified by clinical site and age group
Blinding: Double-blinded
Statistical methods: Intention-to-treat analysis, Kaplan-Meier curves, Cox-proportional hazards models

Results
Participant flow: 373,092 screened, 18,845 enrolled and 16,608 randomized. 331 women initially randomized to unopposed estrogen were unblinded and reassigned to estrogen plus progestin. 42% discontinuation of active treatment; 10.7% crossover from placebo to treatment arm. Eight-year planned follow-up, study terminated early at 5.2 yr.
Baseline data: Mean age: 63.3 yr. Women in the placebo group were more likely to have had a CABG or coronary angioplasty.
Outcomes and estimation: The trial was stopped early when the 10th interim review showed persistent adverse effects in CHD, breast cancer, and the global index outcomes. Hazard ratios with 95% CI were: 1.29 (1.02-1.63) for CHD and 1.26 (1.00-1.59) for invasive breast cancer.

Discussion
Conclusion: "The results indicate that this regimen should not be initiated or continued for primary prevention of CHD."
Limitations: Tested only one regimen, high crossover rates, early stoppage

Funding: National Heat, Lung, and Blood Institute; Wyeth-Ayerst Research

---

Commentary   *Jonathan Soverow, MD, MPH, Resident in Internal Medicine*
The WHI surprised many by showing an increase in CHD, stroke, PE, and invasive breast cancer in healthy women using combined HRT with comparatively minimal benefit in fracture and colorectal cancer reduction. A similar but smaller trial in women with known CHD, the Heart and Estrogen Replacement Study (HERS), showed no cardiovascular benefit to combined HRT [JAMA. 1998;280:605]. A well-designed, large RCT, WHI notably used a weighted index of the first adverse event to quantify the overall risk/benefit balance, rather than relying on mortality rates, where there was no difference. Individual patients and physicians may not weigh these events similarly. Modeling suggested that prolonging the trial would not have captured long-term CHD benefits. And the final, 13-year follow-up of combined therapy in WHI confirmed these trends [JAMA 2013; 310: 1353]. A separate trial in WHI showed no CHD benefit or harm to unopposed estrogen therapy post-hysterectomy [JAMA. 2004;291:1701].

3

FINAL REPORT ON THE ASPIRIN COMPONENT OF THE ONGOING PHYSICIANS' HEALTH STUDY
Steering Committee of the Physicians' Health Study Research Group
New England Journal of Medicine. 1989; 321: 129

Summary: In healthy men older than fifty years of age, low-dose aspirin reduces the risk of first myocardial infarction.

Introduction: Several studies have shown the benefit of aspirin (ASA) in preventing recurrent myocardial infarction (MI), though few have investigated its role in primary prevention of MI.

Objective: "To test a primary-prevention hypothesis [of] whether aspirin in low doses reduces mortality from cardiovascular disease"

Methods
Trial Design: Randomized, US. 2x2 factorial design also investigating the role of beta carotene on primary prevention of cancer.
Participants: Male physicians age 40-84 residing in US. Excluded: history of MI, stroke or transient ischemic attack, cancer, current liver or renal disease, peptic ulcer, or gout; contraindications to ASA; current use of ASA, other platelet-active drugs, NSAIDs, or a vitamin A supplement
Interventions: ASA 325mg QOD vs. placebo QOD
Outcomes: Primary outcome not specified. First MI; first stroke; total cardiovascular deaths
Sample size: 22,071; power calculations not provided
Randomization: Computer-generated list of random numbers
Blinding: Double-blinded
Statistical methods: Intention-to-treat analysis; Statistical methods not well-described

Results
Participant flow: 59,285 willing to participate, 33,223 after exclusion enrolled in 18-week run-in, 22,071 randomized. Five-year follow-up (study terminated early)
Baseline data: No significant differences
Outcomes and estimation: Planned follow-up of 12 years but stopped at 60 months due to demonstrated benefit of ASA; ASA vs. placebo: 139 MI vs. 239 (RR 0.56, p<0.00001, RRR 44%); 119 strokes vs. 98 (RR 1.22, p=0.15); 81 CV deaths vs. 83 (RR 0.96, p=0.87)
Ancillary analyses: Benefit of ASA for MI seen only in age >50 subgroup. No differential effect of ASA when stratified by cholesterol levels, smoking status, diabetes, body mass index or blood pressure
Harms: GI discomfort: ASA 26.1% vs. 25.6% (p=0.45); GI ulcers: ASA 1.5% vs. 1.3% (p=0.08); 'Bleeding problems:' ASA 27% vs. 20.4% (p<0.0001)

Discussion
Conclusion: "This trial of aspirin for the primary prevention of cardiovascular disease demonstrates a conclusive reduction in the risk of MI."
Limitations: Not applicable to women, low rate of events

Funding: National Institutes of Health

Commentary   *Rob McGarrah, MD, Resident in Internal Medicine*
The Physicians' Health Study (PHS) was the largest and most definitive RCT to demonstrate the role of aspirin in primary prevention of MI and still serves as the backbone for society recommendations and guidelines. A recent meta-analysis performed of six large-scale RCT confirmed this benefit in risk reduction of first MI in low-risk healthy individuals [*Lancet* 2009;373:1849]. However, as in PHS, the role of aspirin in prevention of stroke or death remains equivocal. Of note, PHS enrolled only men and event rates were lower than expected (i.e. 'healthy volunteer' phenomenon) hence limiting its generalizability. The risk of bleeding in the aspirin group is significantly higher so this possibility must be weighed against the potential cardiovascular benefits.

MAJOR OUTCOMES IN HIGH-RISK HYPERTENSIVE PATIENTS RANDOMIZED TO ANGIOTENSIN-CONVERTING ENZYME INHIBITOR OR CALCIUM CHANNEL BLOCKER VS DIURETIC (ALLHAT)
The ALLHAT Officers and Coordinators for the ALLHAT Collaborative Research Group
Journal of American Medical Association. 2002; 288: 2981

Summary: Thiazide diuretics are unsurpassed in preventing cardiovascular outcomes with lower risk of heart failure compared to ACEI and CCB in diverse, high risk population.

Introduction: The use of diuretics for blood pressure control declined as newer antihypertensives were developed. Newer agents are effective at preventing cardiovascular disease (CVD) but have not been compared to low-cost diuretics in a randomized controlled trial.

Objective: "To determine whether treatment with a calcium channel blocker or an angiotensin converting enzyme inhibitor lowers the incidence of coronary heart disease or other cardiovascular disease events vs treatment with a diuretic."

Methods
Trial Design: Randomized, multicenter (US and Canada)
Participants: Adults ≥55 with stage 1 or 2 HTN and one other coronary heart disease (CHD) risk factor (74% Medicare or VA beneficiaries)
Interventions: Four arms initially but doxazosin arm discontinued early. Three arms: chlorthalidone (12.5 to 25 mg/day) vs. amlodipine (2.5 mg to 10 mg/day) vs. lisinopril (10 to 40 mg/day). Study drug titrated to goal BP < 140/90, open-label drugs added to step-up treatment at providers' discretion
Outcomes: Primary: fatal or non-fatal CHD; Secondary: all-cause mortality, CVA, combined CHD, combined cardiovascular disease (CVD)
Sample size: 33,357; 83% power to detect a 16% reduction in primary outcome
Randomization: 1.7:1:1 blocked random assignment to three groups; stratified by center
Blinding: Double-blinded
Statistical methods: Intention-to-treat analysis; Kaplan-Meier cumulative event rates, Cox proportional hazards regression

Results
Participant flow: 33,357 recruited, 40-42% completed 5 yr follow-up, 14-15% confirmed mortality in each group
Baseline data: No significant differences
Outcomes and estimation: No difference between the groups in CHD events (chlorthalidone 11.5%, amlodipine 11.3%, lisinopril 11.4%). Amlodipine and lisinopril associated with more heart failure (10.2% and 8.7% vs. 7.7% for chlorthalidone, p<0.001)
Ancillary analyses: Subgroup analyses included gender, race, age, diabetes, and baseline CHD. The findings of equivalency persisted in all groups.
Harms: Increased CVD including heart failure among a doxazosin arm, this arm was terminated early

Discussion
Conclusion: Thiazide diuretics are equivalent or better than ACEI and CCB in preventing CVD and should be considered for first-line antihypertensive medication.
Limitations: BP goals achieved were not equivalent among the study groups. The step-up drugs used excluded three popular study drugs. Unclear if results represent class effect or the medications used in the study

Funding: National Heart, Lung and Blood Institute with medications from AstraZenica, Bristol-Myers Squibb, and Pfizer (who also contributed financially)

Commentary   *Gina Kruse, MD, MS, Resident in Internal Medicine*
The consistency of findings across subgroups and the large numbers make the findings of ALLHAT generalizeable. It is a powerful study with more total cardiovascular events than all prior randomized trials combined. Subsequent studies and meta-analyses have corroborated the results showing non-inferiority of thiazides in preventing cardiovascular outcomes, and lower rates of heart failure, with the exception of the ASCOT trial, which suggested combination CCB /ACEi may be superior to combination beta-blocker / thiazide therapy [Lancet. 2005;366:895-906]. While thiazide diuretic use was associated with diabetes in subsequent analyses of the ALLHAT data, this was not associated with worse cardiovascular outcomes. ALLHAT was an important study in recognizing the non-inferiority of low cost diuretics in reducing cardiovascular events and has influenced prescribing patterns along with JNC7 (Joint National Committee) recommendations that thiazide diuretics be used as first line therapy.

A CONTROLLED TRIAL OF HUMAN PAPILLOMAVIRUS TYPE 16 VACCINE
Koutsky L, Ault K, Wheel C, et al.
New England Journal of Medicine. 2002; 347: 1645

Summary: Human papillomavirus type 16 (HPV-16) vaccination decreases the incidence of HPV-16 infection and HPV-16-associated cervical intraepithelial neoplasia in young women.

Introduction: Infection with HPV-16 is widespread and chronic infection is associated with cervical cancer.

Objective: "To determine whether [HPV-16] vaccine could prevent HPV-16 infection in women."

Methods
Trial Design: Randomized, multicenter (16 centers in the US)
Participants: Non-pregnant women 16- 23 years old with no history of abnormal Pap smear, evidence of current HPV-16 infection, or more than five lifetime male sex partners, and were not immunosuppressed
Interventions: Three doses (day 0, month 2, month 6) of HPV-16 virus-like particle vaccine vs. placebo
Outcomes: Primary: persistent HPV-16 infection as defined by detection of HPV-16 on two or more consecutive visits four or more months apart; demonstration of HPV-16 associated cervical intraepithelial neoplasia (CIN) or cervical cancer on biopsy; or detection of HPV-16 DNA on the visit before being lost to follow-up. Women were seen every 6 months for specimen collection.
Sample size: 2392; 90% power to detect 31 cases of persistent HPV-16 infection
Randomization: Randomized, permuted-block design in 1:1 ratio at each site
Blinding: Double-blinded
Statistical methods: Exact conditional test as measure of vaccine efficacy

Results
Participant flow: 2392 enrolled; 1194 received vaccine and 1198 received placebo. 859 excluded from primary analysis (most commonly due to evidence of HPV-16 infection at enrollment), equal numbers excluded from each group. Median follow-up of 17.4 months after completion of vaccine series
Baseline data: No significant difference. Median age 20, 76% white
Outcomes and estimation: 3.8 (41 cases) vs 0 (0 cases) incidence per 100 woman-years of *persistent* HPV-16 infection and 9 vs 0 cases of HPV-16 associated CIN in placebo versus vaccinated (100% vaccine efficacy; 95% CI 90-100, p<0.001).
Ancillary analyses: 6.3 (68 cases) vs 0.6 (6 cases) incidence per 100 woman-years of *transient* HPV-16 infection in placebo versus vaccinated (91% vaccine efficacy; 95% CI 80-97, no p-value calculated by investigators); 22 vs 22 cases of non-HPV-16 associated CIN in placebo vs vaccinated
Harms: Incidence of adverse events (pain at injection site, fever) was similar in the two groups.

Discussion
Conclusion: HPV-16 vaccination reduces the incidence of persistent HPV-16 infection and HPV-16 associated CIN.
Limitations: The study did not assess vaccine effect on HPV-16 associated cervical cancer.

Funding: Merck Research Laboratories (manufacturers of the HPV-16 vaccine)

Commentary   *Andrew Courtwright, MD, PhD, Resident in Internal Medicine*
This proof-of-concept trial demonstrated that a "cancer vaccine" can be effective; however, it excluded women with a history of abnormal Pap smears, evidence of prior HPV-16 infection, or over five lifetime partners, limiting its generalizability. A study (FUTURE II) of the quadrivalent vaccine, including HPV types 6/11/16/18, showed less vaccine efficacy (17% for high grade CIN) in a population with and without prior infection [NEJM. 2007;356:1915]. To date there has been no evidence to show that HPV vaccine alters the course of HPV infections present before vaccination. Because of the multiplicity of HPV subtypes causing cervical cancer, vaccination does not replace the need for screening, and non-vaccine subtypes may eventually replace the oncological niche of HPV 16 and 18. Nevertheless, efficacy in non-exposed individuals has led to widespread adoption of (non-mandatory) HPV vaccination in the US, beginning at age 11 in women. Subsequent studies have shown efficacy of the quadrivalent HPV vaccine in reducing anal intraepithelial neoplasia and HPV infection in HPV-naïve men [NEJM 2011;364:401].

The Implications Of Regional Variations in Medicare Spending, Part 1: Content, Quality, and Accessibility of Care

Fisher E, Wennberg D, Stukel T, et al.
Annals of Internal Medicine. 2003; 138: 273

Summary: Increased inpatient and specialist care in higher-spending regions account for the majority of regional differences in Medicare spending, but do not augment quality nor accessibility of care

Introduction: Regional differences in Medicare spending exist, but their effect on quality and availability of health care has not been elucidated.

Objective: "To determine whether regions with higher Medicare spending provide better care."

Methods

Trial Design: Cohort Study, consisting of 4 parallel cohorts.

Participants: Medicare enrollees, age 65-99, hospitalized between 1993 and 1995 for hip fracture (n=614,503), colorectal cancer (n=195, 429), myocardial infarction (n=159,393), and a representative sample from the Medicare Current Beneficiary Survey (MCBS) (n=18,190)

Exclusions: A previous hospitalization for the same diagnosis in the preceding year. Enrollment in an HMO

Randomization: Natural randomization approach was used, where end-of-life expenditure index (EOL-EI), the age-sex-race adjusted spending on hospital and physician services for a patient during the last six months of life, served as the random exposure variable. EOL-EI measures regional variation in Medicare spending unrelated to differences in illness or price

Exposure: Based on expenditures for patients in their last 6 months of life, regions were classified into quintiles of expenses incurred. Patients who entered the cohort study after a qualifying event (hip fracture, MI, or colon cancer) were assigned a geographic region based on the HRR in which he/she lived

Outcomes: Content of care (eg. type and frequency of care); quality of care (eg. provision of accepted "best" practices); accessibility of care

Sample size: 987,515

Statistical methods: Logistic or linear regression

Results

Patient Characteristics: Illness levels did not vary significantly across quintiles. African Americans were over-represented in higher–spending regions. Higher spending regions also had a greater number of enrollees in the highest and lowest income levels

Outcomes: Patients in higher-spending quintiles received approximately 60% more care, including more frequent physician visits, specialist consultations, tests, and minor (but not major) procedures as well as an increased use of hospitals (more inpatient days and more days in the intensive care unit). Differences in quality measures were small and inconsistent. Higher spending regions were not associated with better quality of care and in fact, tended to perform poorer on preventive care measures. No significant differences in access to care were found between groups

Harms: None identified

Discussion

Conclusion: Higher-spending regions use more inpatient and specialist-based practice patterns. Increased spending did not improve the quality of or access to care for Medicare enrollees.

Limitations: Studied only 4 disease cohorts. Does not take explicitly into account other differences that may affect health status (ie. disease burden)

Funding: Robert Wood Johnson Foundation and National Institute of Ageing

---

Commentary   *Maria Han, MD, Resident in Internal Medicine*

This study demonstrates that higher levels of Medicare spending in some regions result from the provision of more care but that this additional care does not translate into improved health care quality or access. Critics argue that much of the regional variation in health care spending can be explained by differences in the patient populations between regions, including disease burden and socio-economic factors. This study is the largest conducted on this topic and is generalizable across multiple disease cohorts. Its strength lies in the achievement of "randomization" of treatment groups, as evidenced by similar illness levels across quintiles. This study is limited in its generalizability to other age cohorts and in its lack of prospective recommendations regarding how reductions in health care supply will impact health outcomes or spending.

THE IMPLICATIONS OF REGIONAL VARIATIONS IN MEDICARE SPENDING, PART 2: HEALTH OUTCOMES AND SATISFACTION WITH CARE

Fisher E, Wennberg D, Stukel T, et al.
Annals of Internal Medicine. 2003; 138: 288

Summary: Increased Medicare spending is not associated with improvement in survival, functional status, or patient satisfaction across multiple cohorts with similar illness levels

Introduction Regional differences in Medicare spending exist, but their effect on the health outcomes and satisfaction of care has not been elucidated

Objective: "To determine whether regions with higher Medicare spending achieve better survival, functional status, or satisfaction with care."

Methods
Trial Design: Cohort Study, consisting of 4 parallel cohorts
Participants: Medicare enrollees, age 65-99, hospitalized between 1993 and 1995 for hip fracture (n=614,503), colorectal cancer (n=195,429), myocardial infarction (n=159,393), and a representative sample from the Medicare Current Beneficiary Survey (MCBS) (n=18,190).
Exclusions: A previous hospitalization for the same diagnosis in the preceding year. Enrollment in an HMO
Randomization: Natural randomization approach was used, where end-of-life expenditure index (EOL-EI) served as the random exposure variable. EOL-EI is the age-sex-race adjusted spending on hospital and physician services for a patient during the last six months of life. It intends to measure the component of regional variation in Medicare spending that is unrelated to differences in illness or price
Exposure: Based on EOL-EI, geographic hospital referral regions (HRRs) (n=306) were divided into quintiles of increasing Medicare spending. Patients were assigned to "treatment groups" (one of the quintiles) based on the HRR in which he/she lived
Outcomes: 5-yr mortality rate (all cohorts); change in functional status (MCBS); satisfaction with care (MCBS).

Sample size: 987,515
Statistical methods: Cox proportional hazards regression model; generalized estimating equation methods for the analysis of continuous longitudinal data

Results
Baseline data: Illness levels did not vary significantly across quintiles. African Americans were over-represented in higher quintiles. Both highest and lowest income groups were over-represented in highest quintile
Outcomes and estimation: Quintiles of higher spending were associated with slightly increased mortality. There was no difference in functional status or satisfaction with care across quintiles. Satisfaction of care was higher in the Northeast region than in the South, but this was not related to HRR or level of spending
Harms: None identified

Discussion
Conclusion: This study did not demonstrate any improvement in survival, functional status, or satisfaction of care with higher levels of Medicare spending
Limitations: Unable to determine causality between mortality and treatment differences. Unmeasured confounders, rather than treatment differences, may be the cause of the different mortality rates. The study examined functional status and satisfaction only in the general (MCBS) population sample, not in the disease cohorts

Funding: Robert Wood Johnson Foundation and National Institute of Ageing

---

Commentary   *Maria Han, MD, Resident in Internal Medicine*
This study shows that there is no benefit in mortality, functional status, or satisfaction with care as a result of increased rates of Medicare spending. Similarly to Part 1 of this study, these findings suggest that increased health services and technologies do not necessarily confer population-level health benefits. This study is the largest conducted on this topic and is generalizable across multiple disease cohorts. This study is limited in its ability to instruct how the amount of care offered to a particular patient will affect his/her individual health outcomes. Further, it has been criticized for not sufficiently adjusting for the disease burden of various populations as well as regional price variation. Despite the limitations, this study, also known as the Dartmouth Atlas project, has had a profound affect on health policy.

DOES FREE CARE IMPROVE ADULTS' HEALTH? [THE RAND HEALTH INSURANCE EXPERIMENT]

Brook R, Ware J, Rogers W, et al.
New England Journal of Medicine. 1983; 309: 1426

Summary: With the exception of low income individuals at high risk for poor health, free medical care does not improve health status

Introduction: Patients receiving free care use a third more medical services than patients who share care costs, but it is not known whether increased utilization improves health status

Objective: "Were people who received free medical care, and who thus used more of it, healthier as a result?"

Methods

Trial Design: Randomized, multicenter (US)

Participants: Adults between ages 14 and 61 from families making <$54,000/yr (1982 value) and who were not eligible for Medicare disability insurance

Interventions: One of four categories of insurance: free care vs various cost-sharing plans (individual, intermediate, and catastrophic deductibles)

Outcomes: Health status (self-assessed general health, smoking, weight, cholesterol, diastolic blood pressure, functional far vision, and risk of dying)

Sample size: 3958 people from 2005 families (no power calculation)

Randomization: Random-sampling assignment by family

Blinding: Unblinded

Statistical methods: Regression analysis comparing the health status at study end of individuals with free care vs cost sharing; secondary analysis stratified by family income (low vs high) and initial health (low- vs high-risk for poor health)

Results

Participant flow: 3958 enrolled; 12% from cost sharing and 5% from free care group left study

Baseline data: No significant difference between groups; mean age 33, 88% white

Outcomes and estimation: Visual acuity 20/22 vs 20/22.5 free care vs cost sharing (p<0.05); diastolic pressure 78.5 vs 79.2 free care vs cost sharing (p=0.06); otherwise no difference in health status measures

Ancillary analyses: Low income subjects at high risk for poor health with free care compared to same group with cost sharing had 3.3 mmHg reduction in diastolic pressure and 0.3 fold reduced risk of death (p<0.05)

Harms: No adverse events reported

Discussion

Conclusion: Increased cost of medical care reduced utilization of health care. For the average American, free care and increased use of medical services does not decrease poor health habits (smoking, weight, cholesterol) or improve overall health status. For low income individuals at high risk for poor health, free care improves mortality.

Limitations: There may have been selection bias for although the plans were randomly assigned, people could choose to accept and reject the plan. There were different acceptance rates among the groups. The study authors attempted to investigate the influence of such a bias by looking at health status of all enrollees at the start of the study and no significant differences were found. Could not determine benefit of free care for older individuals and those too disabled to work; these groups were excluded from the study

Funding: United States Department of Health, Education, and Welfare

---

Commentary   *Andrew Courtwright, MD, PhD, Resident in Internal Medicine*

Although the RAND Health Insurance Experiment (HIE) remains the only large trial of insurance cost sharing and health status, it enrolled a relatively young, healthy population at a time when fewer options for treating diseases like hypertension were available, thus limiting the study's generalizability. Nevertheless, results from the HIE have been used to justify various forms of cost-sharing, primarily deductibles, as a standard part of insurance plans as a mechanism to reduce utilization of healthcare and therefore reduce costs for the payer. In 2011, Massachusetts' state-sponsored health care (CommCare) employed a cost sharing method that adjusted for income, in part, because of considerations from the HIE. That cost sharing had no impact on health behaviors like smoking argues against free care creating a "moral hazard," causing individuals to neglect their health.

PATHOLOGIC FINDINGS FROM THE BREAST CANCER SURVEILLANCE CONSORTIUM
Weaver DL, Rosenberg RD, Barlow WE, et al.
Cancer. 2006; 106: 732

Summary: The rate of breast biopsy and diagnosis of carcinoma following screening mammogram was low (1.61% and 0.53% respectively).

Introduction: Breast cancer mortality has declined over the past quarter century, and these changes had been attributable to advances in detection and treatment.

Objective: "To report the histology distribution of benign and malignant outcomes after screening mammography in a large, geographically diverse population of women."

Methods
Study Design: Secondary-data analysis
Participants: Data was included from five population-based cancer and pathology registries from the Breast Cancer Surveillance Consortium (BCSC) that collected both pathology data and cancer registry data of women ages 40-89 who had undergone screening mammograms during the years 1996-2001. Excluded: mammograms were done for non-screening purposes
Interventions and Outcomes:
Mammography: Each mammogram was assigned initial and final Breast Imaging, Reporting, and Diagnosis System Category (BI-RADS) assessments
Pathology and Breast Carcinoma: Included specimens collected within one year after the screening mammogram or before the next screening mammogram if that occurred at < 1 year. The results were classified as benign, ductal carcinoma in situ (DCIS), or invasive carcinoma. Lymph node status and tumor size were obtained for women with invasive carcinoma. Tumor data was compared with data from the Surveillance, Epidemiology, and End Results (SEER) database
Sample size: 1,664,032 screening mammograms from 786,846 women
Randomization: N/A
Blinding: N/A
Statistical methods: Not well-described

Results
Outcomes: Of the 1,664,032 screening mammograms, 26,748 (1.61%) were followed by a subsequent breast biopsy and 8,815 (0.53%) were diagnosed with breast carcinoma. Of those diagnosed with breast carcinoma, 7,143 (81.0%) were invasive carcinomas and the remainder were DCIS. The percent of biopsies classified as DCIS or invasive carcinoma increased with age (p<0.0001) and were more likely if the screening mammogram had been categorized as BI-RADS Category 5. Of those biopsies diagnosed as benign or lobular carcinoma in situ (LCIS) pathology, the breakdown into diagnosis categories is as follows: ductal hyperplasia without atypia (19.6%), fibroadenoma (18.5%), atypical hyperplasia (5.0%), LCIS (0.8%) and other benign (56.1%).
Harms: None identified

Discussion
Conclusion: This study establishes the rates of biopsy and pathology outcomes of those biopsies after undergoing screening mammography.
Limitations: A high number of women (32%) for whom biopsy was recommended after mammogram have no record of biopsy results. Patients within the BCSC may have gone outside of the BCSC health systems for biopsies. These results may underestimate the biopsy rate. Racial and ethnic differences were not taken into account in the study. Differences between tumors detected by screening mammography versus those detected during follow-up were not investigated in the study.

Funding: National Cancer Institute

Commentary   *Lindsay Jubelt, MD, Resident in Internal Medicine*
This study helps to establish expectations for women undergoing screening mammograms by providing the biopsy rate and pathology results of biopsies following screening exams. Mammograms have played an essential role in women's health maintenance for several decades. Early studies showed that screening mammograms reduced the breast cancer mortality rate [Lancet 2002;359:909]. However, recent studies have suggested that much of the decrease in mortality from breast cancer over recent years may be attributable to improvements in treatment strategies rather than from mammogram screening programs [NEJM 2010;363:1203]. Screening mammography is beneficial in certain age groups; however, the benefits may be more modest than what was once thought, and the test is associated with a high rate of false positive results [BMJ 2006;332:689].

EFFECTS OF CLOPIDOGREL IN ADDITION TO ASPIRIN IN PATIENTS WITH ACUTE CORONARY SYNDROMES
WITHOUT ST-SEGMENT ELEVATION (CURE)
The Clopidogrel in Unstable Angina to Prevent Recurrent Events (CURE) Trial Investigators
New England Journal of Medicine. 2001; 345: 494

Summary: Early and long-term administration of clopidogrel reduces the risk of major cardiovascular events in patients with non-ST-elevation acute coronary syndromes but is associated with an increased risk of bleeding.

Introduction: The role of upfront and chronic combined therapy with aspirin and clopidogrel in the treatment of non-ST segment elevation acute coronary syndromes (ACS) is unclear but may have an added protective effect to aspirin alone.

Objective: "To compare the efficacy and safety of the early and long-term use of clopidogrel plus aspirin with those of aspirin alone in patients with acute coronary syndromes and no ST-segment elevation."

Methods
Trial Design: Randomized, multicenter (482 in 28 countries)
Participants: Adults with ischemic EKG changes or elevated cardiac biomarkers but no ST-segment elevation, within 24hrs of symptom onset. Excluded: contraindications to antithrombotic or antiplatelet therapy; high risk of bleeding or CHF; on oral anticoagulants; recent coronary revascularization or GP IIb/IIIa inhibitor use.
Interventions: ASA (75-325mg daily) plus: clopidogrel (300mg PO load, then 75mg daily) vs. placebo
Outcomes: Primary: (1) composite of CV death, nonfatal MI, stroke and; (2) composite of 1st primary outcome or refractory ischemia; secondary: severe ischemia, CHF, revascularization; safety outcomes: major and minor bleeding
Sample size: 12,500; 90% power to detect >16% risk reduction in primary outcomes
Randomization: Concealed from investigators, stratified according to center
Blinding: Double-blinded
Statistical methods: Intention-to-treat analysis; log-rank statistic or chi-square test; Cox regression model

Results
Participant flow: 12,562 enrolled and randomized; 13 lost to follow up (6 clopidogrel, 7 placebo). Twelve-month follow-up.
Baseline data: No significant differences (mean age 64, 62% men)
Outcomes and estimation: First primary composite outcome: reduction in the clopidogrel group (9.3% vs. 11.4%, RR 0.80, p<0.001; NNT=48); similar with second primary outcome (16.5% vs 18.8%, RR 0.86, p<0.001; NNT=44). Rate of each outcome component was lower in the clopidogrel group, with the clearest difference in rates of MI. Lower rates of severe ischemia or recurrent angina in the clopidogrel group
Ancillary analyses: Benefit was seen within 24hrs, preserved over time and across subgroups, including those patients who ultimately require revascularization with PCI.
Harms: Higher risk of minor (NNH=100) and major (NNH=37) bleeding in the clopidogrel group, but no difference in life-threatening bleeding or hemorrhagic stroke. Bleeding after CABG was no different if study medication was held for at least 5d pre-operatively.

Discussion
Conclusion: The addition of clopidogrel to ASA in patients with non-ST segment elevation ACS improved cardiovascular outcomes (reduced MI and recurrent ischemia) but is associated with an increased risk of non-fatal bleeding.
Limitations: Limited to centers with low rates of angiography and revascularization

Funding: Sanofi-Synthelabo, Bristol-Myers Squibb [manufacturers of Plavix (clopidogrel)]

Commentary   *Shweta Motiwala, MD, Resident in Internal Medicine*
Findings from the CURE trial support the early and long-term (up to 12 months) use of clopidogrel in addition to aspirin in the management of non-ST elevation ACS (i.e. UA/NSTEMI). The benefit of clopidogrel was observed in patients who do and do not ultimately undergo coronary revascularization. A subgroup analysis of the CURE trial including patients who underwent PCI – PCI-CURE (Lancet. 2001;358:527) – demonstrated a benefit of pretreatment with clopidogrel prior to the intervention. Because there was a trend toward increased post-operative bleeding when clopidogrel was administered within 5 days of CABG (9.6% vs. 6.3%, RR 1.53, p=0.06), a strategy incorporating clopidogrel in the early management of ACS may prolong the length of stay in patients requiring CABG.

INTENSIVE VERSUS MODERATE LIPID LOWERING WITH STATINS AFTER ACUTE CORONARY SYNDROMES (PROVE-IT)

Cannon CP, Braunwald E, McCabe CH, et al. for the TIMI-22 Investigators
New England Journal of Medicine. 2004; 350: 1495

Summary: Early intensive statin therapy with atorvastatin 80mg immediately after acute coronary syndrome reduces all-cause mortality and cardiovascular events.

Introduction: The use of statins to lower LDL cholesterol reduces the risk of cardiovascular events and death, but the goal and duration of lipid treatment have not been established.

Objective: "To compare the standard degree of LDL cholesterol lowering to approximately 100mg/dL with the use of 40mg of pravastatin daily with more intensive LDL cholesterol lowering to approximately 70mg/dL with the use of 80mg of atorvastatin daily as a mean of preventing death or major cardiovascular events in patients with acute coronary syndrome."

Methods
Trial Design: Multicenter (349 sites in 8 countries US), randomized, non-inferiority
Participants: Adults hospitalized for ACS within prior 10 days; TC <240mg/dL (<200mg/dL if already on lipid lowering therapy). Excluded: life expectancy <2 years, already on statin at 80mg, need to continue fibrates or niacin, on meds that inhibit cytochrome P450-3A4, PCI within 6 mos or CABG within 2 mos, CK elevation unrelated to MI, hepatic disease, Cr > 2.0 mg/dL
Interventions: Pravastatin 40mg (standard) vs atorvastatin 80mg (intensive)
Outcomes: All-cause mortality, MI, stroke, revascularization by PCI or CABG, UA requiring hospitalization. Secondary: death from coronary heart disease, MI, or revascularization
Sample size: 4000; 87% power to detect non-inferiority of pravastatin with 925 events
Randomization: Permuted-block design
Blinding: Double-blind, double-dummy
Statistical methods: Intention-to-treat analysis, Cox proportional-hazards model

Results
Participant flow: 4162 enrolled and randomized; 33% of pravastatin group and 30% of the atorvastatin group withdrew; 8 lost to follow-up
Baseline data: No difference except for higher rate of PAD in pravastatin group (P=0.03). 25% already on statin with median LDL 106
Outcomes and estimation: Median LDL of 95 on pravastatin vs 62 on atorvastatin (P<0.001). Primary event rate at 2 years: 26.3% pravastatin vs 22.4% atorvastatin (RRR 16%, P=0.005). Trend for benefit was significant at 30 days. Secondary endpoint reduced by 25% in atorvastatin group (P<0.001)
Ancillary analyses: RRR 34% among subjects with baseline LDL>125
Harms: Dose decreased in 1.4% pravastatin vs 1.9% atorvastatin due to side effects or LFT abnormalities (P=0.20); transaminitis 1.1% pravastatin vs 3.3% atorvastatin (P<0.001); myalgias or elevated CK 2.7% pravastatin vs 3.3% atorvastatin (P=0.23). No rhabdomyolysis

Discussion
Conclusion: Intensive statin therapy with high-dose atorvastatin to a LDL goal of 70mg/dL after an acute coronary syndrome reduces all-cause mortality and cardiovascular events.
Limitations: Unclear whether the long-term benefit at 2 years is attributable to continued intensive statin therapy vs. early plaque stabilization vs. anti-inflammation in the acute post-ACS period.

Funding: Bristol-Myers Squibb (maker of pravastatin), Sankyo

Commentary   *Mary H. Zhang, MD, Resident in Internal Medicine*
This study and the contemporaneous REVERSAL trial [JAMA 2004;291:1071] established the benefit of intensive statin therapy in ACS and stable CAD. The study was funded by the makers of pravastatin, who based the concept of the trial on the observation that "pleiotropic" effects of statins (e.g. reducing inflammation) may be as important as their lipid lowering; this was clearly refuted in this study and in REVERSAL. While REVERSAL examined atheroma progression by IVUS in patients with stable CAD, PROVE-IT was the first major trial to establish the benefits of atorvastatin 80mg with regard to clinical endpoints. Prior to this study, the National Cholesterol Education Program (NCEP) guidelines specified a goal of LDL<100 for high-risk patients with known coronary disease or diabetes. The findings from this study led to a NCEP-III guideline revision which lowered the LDL goal to 70 among those with "very high risk," defined as known CAD with at least one major risk factor (diabetes, smoking, high TG, or low HDL) or ACS [Circulation 2004; 110:227].

ASPIRIN, HEPARIN, OR BOTH TO TREAT ACUTE UNSTABLE ANGINA

Theroux P, Helene O, McCans J, et al.
New England Journal of Medicine. 1988; 319: 1105

Summary: Heparin and aspirin (alone or in combination) reduce progression to refractory angina and MI compared to placebo but do not change the need for angioplasty or bypass surgery at three-months.

Introduction: Plaque rupture and thrombus formation are key in the progression of unstable angina to myocardial infarction, and optimal medical therapy to prevent progression was not well understood at the time.

Objective: "We tested the usefulness of aspirin... heparin... and a combination of the two in the early management of acute unstable angina pectoris in a double-blind, randomized, placebo-controlled trial involving 479 patients."

Methods

Trial Design: Randomized, multi center, placebo-controlled

Participants: Patients admitted with unstable angina; diagnosis was based on chest pain which worsened with movement or which was present at rest for >20 minutes; EKG changes consistent with ischemia were required as were normal creatine kinase levels. Excluded: regular ASA or Coumadin use, recent angioplasty, recent CABG, age >75 years

Interventions: ASA, heparin bolus plus infusion, both, or placebo

Outcomes: Refractory angina, myocardial infarction, and death

Sample size: 479 patients

Randomization: Not specified

Blinding: Double-blinded

Statistical methods: Intention-to-treat analysis; two-tailed chi square test

Results

Participant flow: 778 enrolled, 299 excluded prior to randomization; 479 randomized

Baseline data: Some differences in artery involved, gender distribution, and cholesterol levels

Outcomes and estimation: Progression to refractory angina was decreased with heparin or ASA +heparin (RR = 0.31, 0.40; p=0.002) and was no different with ASA alone compared to placebo. MI was reduced in all groups compared to placebo (RR = 0.29 with ASA, 0.06 with heparin, 0.12 with combination; p<0.01 all groups). No deaths occurred

Ancillary analyses: After 3 months, CABG or angioplasty were done at similar rates in all 4 groups

Harms: Serious bleeding may be more common w/ ASA + heparin; unclear significance

Discussion

Conclusion: Heparin during acute unstable angina significantly reduces refractory angina and progression to myocardial infarction. The combination of aspirin and heparin was not superior to heparin alone and increased bleeding events.

Funding: Not reported

Commentary   *Ralph DeBiasi, MD, Resident in Internal Medicine*

This was one of the first papers to prospectively compare aspirin and heparin and the combination of the two to placebo in patients with acute unstable angina in the hospital. Importantly, patients on chronic aspirin were excluded from randomization. The trial was halted after the first interim analysis due to clear benefits of heparin. None of the medical regimens changed longer term need for coronary intervention, namely angioplasty or CABG. While low molecular weight heparins were subsequently shown to be superior to unfractionated heparin for *medical* management of higher-risk acute coronary syndromes in some studies [ESSENCE, *N Eng J Med* 1997; 337: 447; *JAMA* 2004; 292: 89.], the value of low molecular weight heparins in early invasive strategies is less clear, particularly in light of higher bleeding risk and difficulty monitoring these agents with invasive therapy.

EARLY INTRAVENOUS THEN ORAL METOPROLOL IN 45,852 PATIENTS WITH ACUTE MYOCARDIAL
INFARCTION: RANDOMISED PLACEBO-CONTROLLED TRIAL (COMMIT)
Chen Z, Xie J, et al for the COMMIT collaborative group.
Lancet. 2005; 366:1622

Summary: In acute myocardial infarction, early use of beta-blockers reduces recurrent infarction and
ventricular dysrhythmias at the cost of increased cardiogenic shock, with no overall difference in mortality or a
composite outcome of death/reinfarction/cardiac arrest.

Introduction Multiple prior studies have shown
that IV and then PO beta-blocker use decreases
mortality in early acute myocardial infarction
(AMI), but most of these studies were performed
prior to widespread use of fibrinolytic therapy.
Thus there is limited/variable use of beta blocker
in AMI despite potential mortality benefit.

Objective: "In acute MI…to assess the balance of
risks and benefits of adding early intravenous then
oral metoprolol to current standard therapies in a
wide range of patients."

Methods
Trial Design: Randomized, multi-center (1250
hospitals in China); 2x2 factorial design also
examining addition of clopidogrel to ASA in AMI
Participants: Patients with ST elevation, left
bundle branch block, or ST depression within 24h
of onset of symptoms of suspected MI. Excluded:
contraindications to study treatment, plan for PCI
Interventions: 5mg IV metoprolol q2-3 min x 3 if
HR>50bpm and SBP>90mmHg, followed by
50mg oral metoprolol, then 200mg controlled-
release metoprolol starting day 2 vs. matching
placebo
Outcomes: Primary: 1) composite of death,
reinfarction, or cardiac arrest; 2) death from any
cause during treatment period. Secondary:
reinfarction, ventricular fibrillation, other cardiac
arrest, cardiogenic shock
Sample size: 45,000; 95% power to detect an
absolute difference of 10% in primary outcome
Randomization: Sequentially numbered sealed
treatment packs prepared centrally
Blinding: Double-blinded
Statistical methods: Intention-to-treat analysis;
log-rank analysis, Kaplan-Meier analysis

Results
Participant flow: 45,852 patients randomized
(22,923 placebo, 22,929 metoprolol); followed
until hospital discharge or 28d
Baseline data: More patients in the control group
received non-study beta-blocker, antiarrythmics,
ACE-I, CCB; more patients in experimental group
received diuretics (statistically significant)
Outcomes and estimation: No difference in
primary composite outcomes of death,
reinfarction, cardiac arrest (9.4% vs. 9.9%, p=0.10)
and death from all causes (7.7% vs. 7.8%, p=0.69).
Increased risk of cardiogenic shock in
experimental group (5% vs. 3.9%, p<0.0001,
NNH=91) especially in first 2d of hospitalization.
Reduction in reinfarction (2% vs. 2.5%, p=0.001,
NNT=229) and ventricular fibrillation (2.5% vs.
3%, p=0.001, NNT=199) in experimental group.
Ancillary analyses: Reduction in death due to
arrhythmia in experimental group (1.7% vs. 2.2%,
p=0.0002)
Harms: As above

Discussion
Conclusion: Due to the increased incidence of
cardiogenic shock, early IV followed by oral
metoprolol use in AMI should not be routinely
recommended for all patients. To prevent reinfarction and ventricular fibrillation, metoprolol
may be started later in the hospital course (~1-2d).
Limitations: None identified

Funding: Sanofi-Aventis and Bristol-Myers
Squibb (manufacturer of clopidogrel), AstraZeneca
(manufacturer of metoprolol), UK Medical
Research Council, British Heart Foundation

Commentary   *Deepa Kumaraiah, MD, MBA Resident in Internal Medicine*
Prior to COMMIT, the benefit of long-term use of beta blockers in MI was clear, but the benefits of early
use were less certain. Two previous systematic reviews had been completed to assess beta-blockers in AMI.
The first (47 RCTs, 14,920 pts) found no difference in early beta blockers use but significant mortality
benefit after 6 weeks [Prog Cardiovasc Dis. 1985; 5: 335]. The second (51 RCTs, 29,260 pts) found no mortality
difference from days 3 to 36 months, but the trials had very few deaths overall [BMJ. 1999; 318:1730].
COMMIT was the first large RCT to address the question of early use of beta-blockers in AMI. It showed
early use reduced the risk of reinfarction and ventricular fibrillation, but increased the risk of cardiogenic
shock and had no mortality benefit. Of note, patients receiving PCI were not included and the exclusion
criteria were operator dependent, making the results more difficult to generalize. Based on these results, it
has lead to a delay of initiating beta blockers in hemodynamically unstable patients and those at increased
risk of cardiogenic shock (age > 70, SBP < 120, HR > 110, and/or Killip class III).

OPTIMAL MEDICAL THERAPY WITH OR WITHOUT **PCI** FOR STABLE CORONARY DISEASE (COURAGE)
Boden W, O'Rourke R, Teo K, et al. for the COURAGE Trial Research Group
New England Journal of Medicine. 2007; 356: 1503

Summary: In patients with stable CAD, optimal medical therapy plus PCI showed no benefit compared to optimal medical therapy alone in terms of death from any cause and non-fatal MI.

Introduction PCI is increasingly common in the treatment of stable CAD despite no proven mortality benefit

Objective: "To determine whether PCI coupled with optimal medical therapy reduces the risk of death and nonfatal myocardial infarction in patients with stable coronary artery disease, as compared with medical therapy alone."

Methods
Trial Design: Prospective randomized controlled trial, multicenter (50 sites in U.S and Canada)
Participants: Adults with stable CAD or Canadian Cardiovascular Society (CCS) class IV angina stabilized by medical management. Excluded: persistent class IV angina, markedly positive stress test, refractory CHF/cardiogenic shock, EF < 30%, revascularization within 6 mo, coronary anatomy not suitable to PCI
Interventions: Optimal medical therapy (OMT) vs. OMT + PCI; OMT = ASA, plavix (if PCI or ASA allergy), simvastatin, long-acting metoprolol and/or amlodipine and/or isosorbide dinitrate, lisinopril or losartan
Outcomes: Composite of all cause mortality and nonfatal MI. Secondary: composite of death, MI, and CVA, hospitalization for UA, QOL, and cost-effectiveness
Sample size: 2270; 85% power to detect an absolute difference of 4.6 % in primary outcome
Randomization: Permuted blocks
Blinding: Unblinded
Statistical methods: Intention-to-treat analysis, Kaplan-Meier method, stratified log-rank statistic, Cox proportional-hazards model, Wilcox rank-sum test, Student's t-test, Cox proportional hazards

Results
Participant flow: 35,539 screened; 2287 patients consented and randomized; 107 in experimental group and 97 in control group lost to follow-up
Baseline data: no significant differences (85% males and 86% Caucasian in both groups)
Outcomes and estimation: Primary outcome occurred in 18.5% of controls vs. 19.0% in intervention arm (p = 0.62). Of note, the PCI+OMT group had statistically less angina at 1 year (P < 0.001) and 3 years (p = 0.02), but not at 5 years. Over mean follow-up of 4.6 years, additional revasc. (PCI or CABG) occurred in 21% of OMT + PCI vs. 32.6% OMT (HR 0.6, P<0.001).
Ancillary analyses: No significant difference in composite of deaths/MI/CVA or in hospitalization for ACS (p = 0.62 and 0.56 respectively)
Harms: None identified

Discussion
Conclusion: As an initial treatment plan, the addition of PCI to optimal medical management did not reduce the incidence of death and nonfatal MI during a follow-up period of 2.5-7.0 years.
Limitations: <10% initially screened patients qualified for enrollment. The study had 85 % males and 86 % Caucasians enrolled limiting generalizability. Also, mostly bare-metal stents were used in the trial.

Funding: Department of Veteran Affairs Cooperative Studies Program, Canadian Institute of Health Research, several pharmaceutical companies gave unrestricted research grants to Dept. of Veteran affairs

Commentary   *Deepa Kumaraiah MD, MBA, Resident in Internal Medicine*
COURAGE was the first large trial to assess PCI vs medical therapy in stable angina during the PCI (vs PTCA) era. It revealed early PCI added to OMT does not decrease the outcome of mortality/nonfatal MI, but had significant limitations, including <10% enrollment and low use of DES. This was a critical trial as PCI rates were rapidly increasing (> 1 million in US in 2004). In the QOL assessment [N Engl J Med 2008; 358:677], the early PCI group had less angina at 3 months and higher QOL at 6 months, but both groups were equal at 36 months. Furthermore, the OMT regimen was very stringent and may not be replicable in the general population. A 2009 meta-analysis (61 trials, 25,000 pt) [Lancet. 2009; 373: 911] revealed similar results with no difference in death or MI between PCI vs OMT as initial management. A 2010 meta-analysis (14 trials, 7800 pt) [Ann Intern Med. 2010; 152: 370] of angina revealed in trials after 2000, no difference in angina with PCI vs OMT initially. Given COURAGE's significant limitations, the ISCHEMIA trial [NCT01471522] was launched to compare OMT and PCI+OMT in 8,000 stable angina patients with positive stress tests and negative CT scans for left main disease.

A COMPARISON OF RATE CONTROL AND RHYTHM CONTROL IN PATIENTS WITH ATRIAL FIBRILLATION (AFFIRM)

Wyse DG, Waldo AL, DiMarco JP, et al
New England Journal of Medicine. 2002; 347: 1825

Summary: In atrial fibrillation, rhythm control is equivalent to rate control with anticoagulation with respect to major clinical outcomes.

Introduction: It was unknown if rhythm control with anti-arrhythmics, cardioversion, and ablation was clinically superior to rate control of atrial fibrillation.

Objective: To "compar[e] the effects of long-term treatment [of AF] with these two strategies"

Methods
Trial Design: randomized, multicenter
Participants: Age >65yrs, recurrent AF, >65 yo or with risk factors for stroke other than age
Interventions: Rhythm control arm: antiarrhythmic (initially) with amiodarone, disopyramide, flecainide, moricizine, procainamide, propafenone, quinidine, sotalol or combinations. Cardioversion, ablation, maze, pacing as necessary. Anti-coagulation continued for 4 mo minimum, but then may be stopped. Rate control with goal HR <80 at rest and <110 with 6min walk, using beta blockers, calcium channel blockers (verapamil and diltiazem), digoxin, or combination. Continuous anticoagulation.
Outcomes: Primary: death. Secondary: composite of death/disabling stroke/disabling anoxic encephalopathy, major bleeding, cardiac arrest
Sample size: 4060; calculation not specified
Randomization: Stratified by center.
Blinding: Unblinded
Statistical methods: Survival analysis with Kaplan-Meier curves and log-rank test for primary intention-to-treat analysis. Cox proportional-hazards for secondary analysis.

Results
Participants: 7401 eligible, 4060 enrolled, 71 withdrew; 26 lost to follow-up. Mean age 69.7 years. Mean follow-up: 3.5yrs. 14.9% crossover from rate to rhythm, 37.5% crossover from rhythm to rate
Baseline data: No significant differences
Outcomes and estimation: More deaths with rhythm vs. rate control group, but non-significant (23.8% vs 21.3%, HR 1.15 [0.99-1.34], p=0.08). Similar results with multivariate analysis of secondary outcomes
Ancillary analyses: Rhythm control led to increased hospitalization (80% vs 73%, p<0.001), torsades de pointes (0.8% vs 0.2%, p=0.07), non-VF/VT cardiac arrest events 0.6% vs. 0.1%, p0.01) and increased drug discontinuation. Stroke rates similar (8.9% vs. 7.4%, NS).

Discussion
Conclusion: Rhythm control offers no mortality or stroke advantages and has higher rates of adverse events (cardiac arrest, dysrhythmia, hospitalization) than rate control.
Limitations: High crossover rates, limited use of anticoagulation in rhythm control group

Funding: NHLBI; Wyeth-Ayerst Laboratories (makers of amiodarone).

Commentary   *Jonathan Soverow, MD, MPH, Resident in Internal Medicine*
This study joined a growing body of evidence, including the similar RACE trial [NEJM 2002; 347: 1834], demonstrating no benefit and significant possible harm to a rhythm control strategy in atrial fibrillation. Perhaps echoing results seen in CAST I and II, much of the harm from rhythm control may have come from the toxicities inherent to anti-arrhythmic drugs, and many have suggested that more benefit may be derived from use of catheter-based rhythm control strategies. Major limitations of AFFIRM include its elderly population, high crossover rates, lack of blinding, and limited use of ablation and anticoagulation in the rhythm control group, as well as relatively short follow-up (3.5 years average). On-treatment analysis of AFFIRM did suggest possible improvements with respect to mortality in patients who sustained sinus rhythm and the DIAMOND trial, [Circulation 2001; 104: 292] which used dofetilide in patients with heart failure, also showed similar benefits in on-treatment analysis, but, as above, intention-to-treat analyses have not demonstrated improved major clinical outcomes with use of anti-arrhythmic pharmacotherapy.

AMIODARONE OR AN IMPLANTABLE CARDIOVERTER-DEFIBRILLATOR FOR CONGESTIVE HEART FAILURE (SCD-HeFT)

Bardy GH, Lee KL, Mark DB, et al.
New England Journal of Medicine. 2005; 352: 225

Summary: Implantable cardioverter defibrillator use decreases mortality in patients with NYHA Class II CHF of both ischemic and non-ischemic etiology, whereas amiodarone is no better than placebo.

Introduction: Patients with CHF are at risk for sudden cardiac death (SCD) due to arrhythmia. The evidence for amiodarone and implantable cardioverter defibrillator (ICD) therapy to suppress arrhythmia was limited to small trials.

Objective: "To evaluate the hypothesis that amiodarone or conservatively programmed shock-only single-lead ICD would decrease the risk of death from any cause in a broad population of patients with mild-to-moderate heart failure."

Methods

Trial Design: Randomized, partially-blinded, multi-center (US & Canada)
Participants: Adults with chronic, stable CHF NYHA Class II-III (ischemic or non-ischemic) with LVEF≤35%. Excluded: history of non-ischemic VT/VF; unexplained syncope in preceding 5 yrs; expected heart transplant; contraindication to amiodarone; AF likely to require amiodarone or AV nodal ablation; mechanical prosthetic valve; Class I or III antiarrhythmic therapy; PPM
Interventions: Conventional medical therapy plus: placebo vs. amiodarone vs. ICD
Outcomes: Death from any cause (primary)
Sample size: 2521; 90% power to detect 25% reduction in death from any cause by amiodarone or ICD therapy vs. placebo
Randomization: Permuted-block randomization with stratification according to clinical site, cause of CHF and NYHA class
Blinding: Blinded for medication, not ICD
Statistical methods: Intention-to-treat; Kaplan-Meier survival curves; log-rank tests; Cox proportional-hazards model

Results

Participant flow: 2521 patients; 847 placebo, 845 amiodarone, 829 ICD; none lost to follow-up
Baseline data: No significant differences, except more patients on BB at end of follow-up in ICD group; median EF 25%; 75-95% compliance with medical therapy in both groups; median follow-up 2yrs
Outcomes and estimation: Amiodarone no better than placebo. Decreased risk of death with ICD therapy – HR 0.77(0.62-0.92; p=0.007), RRR 23%, ARR 7.2% at 5 yrs compared to placebo
Ancillary analyses: Amiodarone group had 44% relative increase in mortality in NYHA class III compared to placebo (HR 1.44 [1.05-1.97]). ICD therapy was better for NYHA class II (RRR 46%, ARR 11.9% in 5-yr mortality) but had no benefit in NYHA class III.
Harms: Amiodarone group had increased rates of tremor and hypothyroidism compared to placebo. ICD complication rate (requiring surgical correction, hospitalization, or new and unanticipated drug therapy) was 5% at implantation and 9% afterwards.

Discussion

Conclusion: Amiodarone does not improve survival in patients with mild-to-moderate systolic CHF. Simple, shock-only ICD therapy improves survival beyond state-of-the-art drug therapy in patients with NYHA Class II CHF, but not in NYHA Class III CHF.
Limitations: Strict programming of ICD (shock-only therapy); cost of ICD

Funding: NHLBI, Medtronic, Wyeth-Ayerst Laboratories, Knoll Pharmaceuticals

---

Commentary   *Fernando M. Contreras, M.D., Resident in Internal Medicine*

SCD-HeFT confirmed that anti-arrhythmic drugs such as amiodarone are not effective for the primary prevention of SCD. Relative to prior ICD trials (including MADIT and MADIT II), this trial explores the benefits of ICD therapy beyond ischemic cardiomyopathy. The mortality benefit was clear, particularly in those patients with NYHA Class II CHF and LVEF≤30%. This benefit was similar in both ischemic and non-ischemic patients. Interestingly, ICD implantation did not confer a mortality benefit in NYHA Class III patients, though the authors argue that this therapy should not be withheld from Class III patients given the mortality benefit seen in preceding trials (MADIT II, DEFINITE). Amiodarone had no survival benefit when compared to placebo and, in fact, was associated with increased mortality in those with NYHA class III CHF. Based on this and similar studies, the 2008 ACC/AHA/HRS Guidelines for Device Therapy recommend ICD implantation in patients with EF<35% and NYHA Class II-III heart failure.

PROPHYLACTIC IMPLANTATION OF A DEFIBRILLATOR IN PATIENTS WITH MYOCARDIAL INFARCTION AND REDUCED EJECTION FRACTION (MADIT II)
Moss AJ, Zareba W, Hall J, et al. for the MADIT II Investigators
New England Journal of Medicine. 2002; 346: 877

Summary: Implantable cardioverter-defibrillator implantation improves survival in patients with prior MI and LV dysfunction (ejection fraction ≤30%).

Introduction: Patients with prior MI and subsequent LV dysfunction are at risk of arrhythmia-related sudden cardiac death (SCD).

Objective: "To evaluate the potential survival benefit of a prophylactically implanted defibrillator (in the absence of electrophysiological testing to induce arrhythmias) in patients with a prior myocardial infarction and a left ventricular ejection fraction of 0.30 or less."

Methods
Trial Design: Randomized, multi-center (71 centers in US, 5 in Europe)
Participants: Adults with prior MI, LVEF≤30%. Excluded: FDA-approved indication for implantable cardioverter-defibrillator (ICD), NYHA Class IV, coronary revascularization in the preceding 3 mos, MI within the preceding month, advanced cerebrovascular disease, childbearing age not on contraception, non-cardiac condition with high risk of death during the trial
Interventions: ICD plus conventional medical therapy vs. conventional medical therapy only
Outcomes: Primary: death from any cause
Sample size: 1232; 95% power to detect 38% reduction in 2yr mortality
Randomization: 3:2 ICD:conventional therapy
Blinding: Unblinded
Statistical methods: Intention-to-treat; Cox proportional-hazards regression model; Kaplan-Meier survival curves

Results
Participant flow: 1232 enrolled and randomized; 54 crossovers (equal between groups); 3 lost to follow up but alive within six months before trial completion. Average follow-up 20mos
Baseline data: No significant differences; mean EF 23±5%
Outcomes and estimation: ICD superior to conventional therapy, with 31% RRR of death from any cause in the ICD group (HR 0.69 [0.51-0.93], p=0.016). Kaplan-Meier survival difference first detected at 9 mos (p=0.007). Mortality RRR: 12% at 1 yr, 28% at 2 yrs and 28% at 3 yrs; ARR 6%, NNT=17
Ancillary analyses: No difference in outcomes in subgroup analyses by age, sex, EF, NYHA class, QRS duration or comorbidities
Harms: 13 lead complications (1.8%), 5 non-fatal infections requiring surgical intervention (0.7%). Patients with ICD had a 5% higher incidence of new or worsened CHF (p=0.09).

Discussion
Conclusion: ICD implantation improves survival in patients with prior MI and advanced LV dysfunction.
Limitations: Cost of ICD implantation to the health care system is substantial. Back-up ventricular pacing may impair LV function, contributing to new or worsened CHF.

Funding: Research grant – Guidant (manufacturer of the ICD used in the study), St. Paul, Minn, to the University of Rochester School of Medicine and Dentistry

Commentary   *Fernando M. Contreras, M.D., Resident in Internal Medicine*
MADIT-II was the first primary prevention ICD trial to eliminate the EP study as an inclusion criteria, which may account for the reduced survival benefit seen in this study compared to prior studies. Despite the survival benefit associated with ICD therapy, the need for optimal medical therapy (BB, ACEI, statin) after MI cannot be overemphasized. Post-hoc analyses of MADIT-II demonstrated improved outcomes in those on BB therapy, with less risk of ventricular tachycardia/fibrillation requiring ICD discharge [Am J Cardiol 2005;96:691]. As a result of this trial and others, the 2008 ACC/AHA/HRS Guidelines for Device Therapy recommend ICD implantation in post-MI patients with EF<35% and NYHA Class I or EF<35% and NYHA Class II/III. In practice, post-MI patients are followed with TTE at ~3mos as early implantation may not result in benefit (see DINAMIT trial, page 19).

PROPHYLACTIC USE OF AN IMPLANTABLE CARDIOVERTER-DEFIBRILLATOR AFTER ACUTE
MYOCARDIAL INFARCTION (DINAMIT)
Hohnloser SH, Kuck KH, Dorian P, et al.
New England Journal of Medicine 2004; 351:2481

Summary: Implantation of a cardioverter defibrillator within 40 days of acute MI does not reduce all-cause mortality.

Introduction: Ventricular tachyarrythmias are a common cause of mortality following acute MI and prior studies have shown a benefit to prophylactic ICD implantation.

Objective: "To test whether prophylactic implantation of an implantable cardioverter-defibrillator (ICD) would reduce mortality in survivors of a recent myocardial infarction who are at high risk for ventricular arrhythmias."

Methods
Trial Design: Randomized, multicenter (12 countries, most centers in Canada and Germany)
Participants: Patients with MI within the preceding 6-40 days, LVEF ≤ 0.35, and impaired cardiac autonomic function (depressed HR variability or elevated 24-hr HR on Holter). Excluded: Symptomatic CHF, limited life expectancy due to non-cardiac disease, CABG or 3-vessel PCI for qualifying MI, on heart transplant list, PPM, other qualification for ICD, poor compliance
Interventions: Medical management vs medical management + ICD
Outcomes: All-cause mortality (primary); death from arrhythmia (secondary)
Sample size: 525; 80% power to detect a 10% absolute difference in mortality
Randomization: Central randomization by coordinating center, stratified by clinical center
Blinding: Unblinded (central committee blinded when reviewing cause of death)
Statistical methods: Intention-to-treat; Kaplan-Meier and Mantel-Haenszel tests

Results
Participant flow: 674 enrolled, 332 randomized to ICD (6% refused implantation) and 342 to control. At 30 mos, 81 in ICD group and 88 in control group were lost to follow-up
Baseline data: Amiodarone prescribed in 8% of ICD group and 13.5% of control group (p=0.04)
Outcomes and estimation: No difference in all-cause mortality at 30 mos (HR 1.08, p=0.66). 12 deaths due to arrhythmia in the ICD group vs 29 in the control group (HR 0.42, p=0.009), though this was offset by more non-arrhythmic deaths in the ICD group (HR 1.75, p=0.02)
Ancillary analyses: In both groups, ~78% of non-arrhythmic deaths were cardiovascular in nature
Harms: In-hospital device-related complications (lead displacement, pneumothorax, inappropriate shocks) occurred in 25 patients with ICD therapy

Discussion
Conclusion: Prophylactic ICD implantation after recent MI reduces arrhythmic but increases non-arrhythmic death, resulting in no overall survival benefit.
Limitations: Impaired HR variability may not be a surrogate marker for those at high risk of arrhythmic death; differential use of amiodarone between the two groups; high loss to follow-up

Funding: St. Jude Medical (makers of ICD)

Commentary   *Aarti Asnani, MD, Resident in Internal Medicine*
As the first major randomized trial to examine ICD implantation following acute MI, DINAMIT represents an important contribution to the literature on appropriate indications for ICD therapy. As expected, ICD implantation reduced the rate of arrhythmic death. Surprisingly, all-cause mortality was unchanged. This finding was subsequently confirmed in a retrospective analysis of MADIT II [Circulation 2004; 109:1082] as well as in IRIS [NEJM 2009; 361:1427], which randomized nearly 900 patients with acute MI and reduced EF to ICD therapy or medical management. The reason for increased non-arrhythmic deaths in the ICD group remains unclear and requires further study. The results of DINAMIT and IRIS have been incorporated into the Centers for Medicare and Medicaid Services (CMS) reimbursement structure as well as the ACC/AHA/HRS guidelines. Thus, ICD implantation is recommended no sooner than 40 days (and in practice often 3 months) following acute MI.

THE EFFECT OF CARDIAC RESYNCHRONIZATION ON MORBIDITY AND MORTALITY IN HEART FAILURE (CARE-HF)

Cleland JG, Daubert JC, Erdmann E, et al.
New England Journal of Medicine. 2005; 352: 1539

Summary: In patients with NYHA Class III or IV heart failure and mechanical dyssynchrony, cardiac resynchronization decreases morbidity and mortality.

Introduction: Many patients with HF have prolonged myocardial activation and subsequent cardiac dyssynchrony. In these patients, cardiac resynchronization therapy (CRT) was shown in previous studies to decrease symptoms and improve exercise capacity, quality of life and LV function.

Objective: "We analyzed the effects of cardiac resynchronization on the risk of complications and death among patients who were receiving standard medical therapy for moderate or severe heart failure and cardiac dyssynchrony."

Methods
Trial Design: RCT, multicenter, international (82 European centers)
Participants: ≥18 years w/ CHF for ≥6 weeks w/ NYHA III or IV despite standard therapy, LVEF <35%, LVEDD ≥30mm and QRS≥120
Interventions: Medtronic InSync III Device, atrial based, biventricular stimulation, backup rate of 60 and AV delay optimized with echo
Outcomes: Composite death from any cause or hospitalization for CV event. Secondary: death from any cause, death from any cause or hospitalization with worsening HF
Sample size: 813; 80% power to detect 14% relative reduction or 5.7% absolute reduction in event rate
Randomization: Stratified by NYHA class
Blinding: Not blinded
Statistical methods: Intention-to-treat analysis; Kaplan-Meier, Cox proportional-hazard models, Fisher's exact test

Results
Participant flow: 813 patients enrolled, 404 randomized to medical therapy and 409 to medical therapy plus resynchronization, followed for a mean of 29.4 months
Baseline data: No significant differences
Outcomes: In control group, 55% met primary endpoint (combined death or unplanned hospitalization) compared to 39% in resynchronization group, (HR 0.63, p<0.001)
Ancillary analyses: In control group, 30% met secondary endpoint of death from any cause compared to 20% in resynchronization group, (HR 0.64, p<0.001). 47% in control and 29% in resynchronization group met "death or unplanned hospitalization with worsening HF" endpoint, (HR 0.54, p<0.001). 33% of control and 18% of resynchronization patients met "unplanned hospitalization with worsening HF" endpoint, (HR 0.48, p<0.001). Resynchronization patients had less severe symptoms per NHYA class score, Minnesota Living with HF score
Harms: One device related death in each group; lead displacement, coronary sinus dissection, pocket erosion, pneumothorax, and device related infections

Discussion
Conclusion: "In patients with heart failure and cardiac dyssynchrony, cardiac resynchronization improves symptoms and the quality of life and reduces complications and the risk of death."
Limitations: Limited to severe HF

Funding: Medtronic Corporation

Commentary   Lauren Gray Gilstrap, MD, Resident in Internal Medicine
This study randomly assigned 813 patients with NYHA III or IV HF, EF<35% and QRS>120 to resynchronization therapy with biventricular pacing in addition to medical therapy versus medical therapy alone. The patients were followed for an average of 29 months. Patients with resynchronization had a reduction in all cause death and hospitalization from a CV cause. This reduction was seen in all groups and did not vary based on age, sex, SBP, LVEF, QRS or medications. Interestingly, the study also showed a reduction in BNP of 225pg/mL at 3 months and of 1122 pg/mL at 18 months – an observation which merits additional investigation. The mortality benefit was due primarily to a reduction in worsening HF, rather than a reduction in lethal arrhythmias. The COMPANION study showed that while resynchronization therapy resulted in a 24% reduction in all cause mortality, resynchronization plus a defibrillator resulted in a 43.4% reduction in mortality [NEJM 2004; 350:2140].

THE EFFECT OF SPIRONOLACTONE ON MORBIDITY AND MORTALITY IN PATIENTS WITH SEVERE
CONGESTIVE HEART FAILURE (RALES TRIAL)
Pitt B, Zannad F, Remme WJ, et al.
New England Journal of Medicine. 1999;341:709

Summary: In patients with severe heart failure, addition of spironolactone to standard therapy reduces
morbidity and mortality.

Introduction: Aldosterone causes Na retention,
Mg/K wasting, and sympathetic, baroreceptor and
arterial wall dysfunction. Aldosterone-receptor
blockers (e.g. spironolactone) historically were
avoided in HF out of concern for hyperkalemia
and because ACE inhibitors suppress aldosterone
production.

Objective: "To test the hypothesis that daily
treatment with 25mg of spironolactone would
significantly reduce the death from all causes
among patients who had severe heart failure."

Methods
Trial Design: Randomized, placebo-controlled,
multicenter (195 centers in 15 countries)
Participants: Adults with LVEF <35% and
NYHA III or IV. Excluded: Valvular disease,
congenital heart disease, unstable angina, hepatic
failure, cancer, pre/post-transplant, Cr>2.5 or
K>5
Interventions: Spironolactone 25mg daily vs.
placebo
Outcomes: Death from all causes. Secondary:
death from cardiac cause, hospitalization from
cardiac cause, change in NYHA class
Sample size: 1663; 90% power to detect a 17%
difference between treatment groups
Randomization: Not specified
Blinding: Double blinded
Statistical methods: Intention-to-treat analysis;
Kaplan-Meier, log-rank test, Cox proportional-
hazards regression model

Results
Participant flow: 1663 patients underwent
randomization - 841 in placebo group, 822 in
spironolactone group; 200 in placebo group and
214 in spironolactone group stopped due to
adverse events/lack of response
Baseline data: No significant differences
Outcomes and estimation: Mean follow-up 24
mos; 386 deaths (46%) in placebo group and 284
deaths (35%) in spironolactone group,
representing a 30% reduction in the risk of death,
(p <0.001)
Ancillary analyses: 30% reduction (RR 0.7;
p<0.001) in hospitalization from cardiac causes
with spironolactone; 32% reduction (RR 0.68;
p<0.001) in combined end point of
death/hospitalizations from cardiac cause with
spironolactone
Harms: No differences in sodium, BP, or HR
between groups; median Cr and K did not change
during first year; median Cr later increased 0.05
and K increased 0.3 which was significantly
different but not clinically relevant. Gynecomastia
occurred in 6.9% of men taking spironolactone

Discussion
Conclusion: Spironolactone decreases overall and
cardiovascular mortality as well as cardiac-related
hospitalization in patients with severe systolic HF
already on ACEI.
Limitations: The study population was confined
to patients with advanced HF.

Funding: Searle (makers of Aldactone)

Commentary   *Lauren Gray Gilstrap, MD, Resident in Internal Medicine*
This study supports the efficacy and safety of spironolactone in severe HF when added to traditional
pharmacologic therapy at the time (ACE inhibitors, Lasix and/or digoxin). This was a well designed,
double-blind, placebo-controlled, randomized trial which enrolled over 1,600 patients. The benefits of
spironolactone were first evident by 3 months and continued for the entire 24 months. The study was
stopped after 24 months of follow up because of a significant (30%) reduction in overall mortality with
spironolactone in both ischemic and non-ischemic CHF patients. Additional research has suggested that
the mortality benefits may have been due to a decrease in ventricular arrhythmias. Complications from
hyperkalemia were rare in this study, which may be attributable to very close monitoring of potassium
homeostasis as well as careful patient selection (all patients in this study had Cr<2.5 and K<5). Potassium
should be very carefully monitored after starting aldosterone blockade. As suggested by the recent trial
EMPHASIS-HF, the benefits of aldosterone antagonism may also extend to patients with less symptomatic
(NYHA II) HF as well [NEJM 2011; 364:11].

COMPARISON OF CARVEDILOL AND METOPROLOL ON CLINICAL OUTCOMES IN PATIENTS WITH CHRONIC HEART FAILURE IN THE CARVEDILOL OR METOPROLOL EUROPEAN TRIAL (COMET): RANDOMISED CONTROLLED TRIAL
Poole-Wilson P, Swedberg K, Cleland J, et al. for the COMET investigators
Lancet.2003;362: 7

Summary: Carvedilol improves survival compared to metoprolol tartrate in patients with chronic heart failure.

Introduction: Certain beta-blockers have been shown to reduce mortality in chronic HF. Studies suggest that carvedilol may improve outcomes compared to metoprolol because of its more comprehensive adrenergic receptor blockade.

Objective: "To compare directly the effects of carvedilol and metoprolol tartrate on mortality and morbidity in patients with mild to severe heart failure from left ventricular systolic dysfunction."

Methods
Trial Design: Randomized, multicenter (341 sites in 15 European countries)
Participants: Adults with HF (NYHA II-IV) and cardiovascular admission within 2 yrs, on stable ACEI and diuretic therapy unless contraindicated, EF <35%. Excluded: IV inotropes, calcium channel blockerss, amiodarone, class I antiarrhythmics; ACS, recent revascularization or CVA; uncontrolled HTN; valvular disease or VT; systemic disease with reduced life expectancy.
Interventions: Carvedilol 3.125mg BID (target dose 25mg BID) or metoprolol tartrate 5mg BID (target dose 50mg BID)
Outcomes: All-cause mortality and composite of all-cause mortality or all-cause admission
Sample size: 3029; powered to detect 20% reduction in mortality, 15% reduction in mortality or admission
Randomization: Concealed from investigators; permuted blocks by center
Blinding: Double-blind
Statistical methods: Intention-to-treat analysis; log-rank test without stratification, Cox proportional hazards model, survival analysis

Results
Participant flow: 3029 enrolled and randomized; 5 lost to follow-up, 28 withdrew consent to further follow-up
Baseline data: No significant differences
Outcomes and estimation: All-cause mortality was significantly lower in the carvedilol group (34% vs. 40%, p=0.0017), an effect which was consistent across all predefined subgroups. No significant difference in the composite endpoint
Harms: Similar adverse events in both groups, most commonly bradycardia and hypotension

Discussion
Conclusion: In patients with chronic HF optimally treated with ACEI and diuretics, carvedilol confers a mortality benefit compared to metoprolol tartrate.
Limitations: Possible effect of underdosing metoprolol; use of metoprolol tartrate rather than succinate, which was the more effectively studied and longer-acting formulation of metoprolol

Funding: Hoffmann La Roche and GlaxoSmithKline

___

Commentary   *Shweta Motiwala, MD, Resident in Internal Medicine*
Beta-blockers have been shown to reduce mortality in patients with chronic CHF, specifically B1-selective bisoprolol (CIBIS-I) and metoprolol succinate (MERIT-HF), as well as non-selective B1/B2/α1-blocking carvedilol (COPERNICUS, US-Carvedilol). COMET was the first head to head comparison of two B-blocking agents with differing pharmacological profiles. It is adequately powered, with inclusion and exclusion criteria that are similar to other comparable trials, making its conclusions generalizable to most patients with symptomatic heart failure. Its major limitation, acknowledged by the authors, is that it does not address the possibility that metoprolol succinate (used in MERIT-HF) may be superior to metoprolol tartrate used in COMET. The B_1-adrenoceptor blocking activity of metoprolol tartrate (assessed by a decrease in heart rate) was less than with carvedilol in COMET over the first 16 months of the trial and less than that observed in previous mortality studies with metoprolol succinate, suggesting that the dosing of metoprolol tartrate was not optimal in COMET.

RANDOMIZED TRIAL OF CHOLESTEROL LOWERING IN 4444 PATIENTS WITH CORONARY HEART
DISEASE: THE SCANDINAVIAN SIMVASTATIN SURVIVAL STUDY (4S)
Scandinavian Simvastatin Survival Study Group
Lancet 1994;344:1383

Summary: Simvastatin therapy is beneficial for secondary prevention of cardiovascular events and mortality in
a population of patients with known coronary heart disease.

Introduction: Although cholesterol is known to
play a role in atherosclerosis, it was unclear
whether lowering cholesterol improves mortality in
patients with coronary heart disease (CHD).

Objective: "To evaluate the effect of cholesterol
lowering with simvastatin on mortality and
morbidity in patients with CHD."

Methods
Trial Design: Randomized, multicenter (94
centers in Scandinavia)
Participants: 4444 patients aged 35-70 with
angina or prior MI and total cholesterol (TC) 5.5-
8.0 mmol/L (213-309 mg/dl) on a lipid-lowering
diet. Excluded: planned angioplasty or CABG, MI
in preceding 6 mos, antiarrhythmic therapy, CHF
requiring diuretics, persistent AF,
hemodynamically significant valvular disease,
history of CVA
Interventions: Simvastatin 20 mg qhs or placebo;
simvastatin dose range 10-40 mg for target TC 3-
5.3 mmol/L (116-205 mg/dl)
Outcomes: Primary: all-cause mortality.
Secondary: major coronary events; any coronary
event, death from any atherosclerotic event,
incidence of coronary revascularization, hospital
admission for acute CHD event
Sample size: 4400; 95% power to detect 30%
reduction in total mortality
Randomization: Not explained; stratified by
clinical site and prior MI
Blinding: Double-blinded
Statistical methods: Intention-to-treat; logrank
test, Cox regression model

Results
Participant flow: 7027 enrolled, 2583 excluded;
4444 randomized; 13% in placebo group and 10%
in statin group discontinued treatment; < 1%
cross-over
Baseline data: No significant differences
Outcomes and estimation: Statin group
demonstrated favorable changes in cholesterol
levels (-25% in TC, -35% in LDL, and +8% in
HDL). All-cause mortality at 5 years was 12% in
placebo group and 8% in statin group (RR 0.7,
P=0.0003)
Ancillary analyses: 34% relative risk reduction
for major coronary events with statin (P<0.00001);
replicated in subset analysis for women and age ≥
60 years
Harms: Same rate of discontinuation and cancer
in both groups; 1 case of rhabdomyolysis in statin
group, few asymptomatic CK and LFT elevations
with statin

Discussion
Conclusion: In patients with known CHD,
simvastatin therapy decreases mortality.
Limitations: Underpowered to detect mortality
difference in women (19% of cohort)

Funding: Merck Research Laboratories,
manufacturer of Zocor (simvastatin)

Commentary   *Aarti Asnani, MD, Resident in Internal Medicine*
The 4S study demonstrated the now well-accepted benefits of statin therapy for secondary prevention in
patients with known CHD. On average, lipid levels in this study were higher than those seen in our
patients today, and many patients with other cardiovascular comorbidities (CHF, persistent AF, etc.) were
excluded from the study. However, the robust effect of statin therapy observed in the study population
suggests that the results may be generalizable to all patients with CHD. This paper forms the cornerstone
of the Adult Treatment Panel (ATP) III guidelines, which recommend aa LDL goal of < 100 mg/dl in
CHD patients. Subsequent studies have demonstrated the benefits of lowering cholesterol to < 70 mg/dl
in patients with known CHD. According to the most recent ACC/AHA guidelines, a more aggressive
approach is reasonable in this high-risk population.

ROSUVASTATIN TO PREVENT VASCULAR EVENTS IN MEN AND WOMEN WITH ELEVATED C-REACTIVE
PROTEIN (JUPITER)
Ridker PM, Danielson E, Fonseca FAH, et al.
New England Journal of Medicine 2008; 359:2195

Summary: In healthy patients with elevated C-reactive protein and normal lipids, rosuvastatin as primary prevention reduced cardiovascular events at 2 years.

Introduction: C-reactive protein (CRP) is a marker of inflammation, and elevated levels predict adverse cardiovascular outcomes. Since statins lower CRP, the authors hypothesized that lowering CRP with a statin could reduce cardiac events.

Objective: "To investigate whether treatment with rosuvastatin, 20 mg daily, as compared with placebo, would decrease the rate of first major cardiovascular events."

Methods
Trial Design: Randomized, placebo-controlled trial in 26 countries
Participants: Men >50 and women >60 without a history of cardiovascular disease, LDL <130 and CRP >2.0, who were not on a statin
Interventions: Rosuvastatin 20 mg daily vs. placebo
Outcomes: First major cardiovascular event (MI, stroke, hospitalization for unstable angina, peripheral arterial intervention, or death from any cardiovascular event)
Sample size: 17,802; powered to detect reduction in primary end point with 90% power.
Randomization: Interactive voice-response system, stratified by center
Blinding: Double-blinded
Statistical methods: Intention-to-treat analysis. Originally designed to run until 520 end points were reached to achieve 90% power to detect 25% reduction in end points

Results
Participant flow: 89,890 people screened of which 17,802 were enrolled
Baseline data: No differences (all with LDL <130, CRP >2.0); 38% women, 25% Hispanic or Black, 41.4% with metabolic syndrome
Outcomes and estimation: Terminated at first interim analysis at 1.9 years; 142 events in statin group and 251 in placebo group (HR 0.56, p <0.00001)
Ancillary analyses: Subgroup analyses yielded similar results. The lowest risk individuals (low BMI, low LDL, non-smokers) had similar benefit and hazard ratios
Harms: No differences in muscle weakness, LFT elevations, GFR reductions. A higher rate of new-onset diabetes mellitus was noted with randomization to rosuvastatin

Discussion
Conclusion: Rosuvastatin reduced rates of a first major cardiovascular event and death from any cause in healthy patients who did not have hyperlipidemia but did have elevated CRP.
Limitations: Excluded people with low levels of CRP; early stoppage, limiting analysis of longer-term effects

Funding: Astra Zeneca (makers of Crestor/rosuvastatin)

Commentary *Ralph DeBiasi, MD, Resident in Internal Medicine*
While inflammatory markers such as CRP are known to be predictive of cardiovascular risk, it was not known whether treating healthy individuals with a statin would prevent cardiovascular events. This trial demonstrated that in healthy subjects with relatively normal cholesterol, using a statin prevented cardiovascular events and lowered all-cause mortality. CRP may reflect global cardiovascular risk, but it is possible that CRP may be indirectly involved in the mechanism by which statins reduce inflammation and cardiac risk. Notably, there was a significant increase in new onset, physician-reported diabetes in the rosuvastatin group. Cost-effectiveness of putting these relatively healthy patients on a statin is not known. Since JUPITER was stopped at 2 years with the number needed to treat imputed on full enrollment, the benefit seen may be overestimated. At present, there is no consensus regarding initiating a statin in patients meeting the profile of the JUPITER study (low LDL, elevated CRP).

CD4 COUNT-GUIDED INTERRUPTION OF ANTIRETROVIRAL TREATMENT (SMART)

El-Sadr WM, Lundgren JD, Neaton JD, et al. for the SMART Study Group
New England Journal of Medicine. 2006; 355: 2283

Summary: Structured interruptions of antiretroviral treatment increases mortality and opportunistic infections without reducing adverse events.

Introduction: Antiretroviral therapy (ART) provides substantial morbidity and mortality benefit to subsets of HIV+ patients. However, the effectiveness of long-term ART can be limited by adverse events including side effects of drugs, problems with adherence and ensuing viral resistance, and burgeoning cost.

Objective: "To compare a treatment strategy of episodic use of ART according to CD4 count with continuous ART."

Methods
Trial Design: Randomized, multicenter
Participants: HIV+ aged > 13yrs with CD4 counts >350 cells/mm^3. Eligibility not affected by current or prior ART. Excluded: Pregnant, breastfeeding
Interventions: Interrupted (drug conservation-DC) ART (start ART if CD4 < 250 or opportunistic infections (OIs) or CD4 lymphs < 15%; stop ART once CD4 >350) vs. continuous (viral suppression-VS) ART
Outcomes: Primary: new or recurrent OIs or death from any cause. Secondary: major cardiovascular, renal or hepatic disease.
Sample size: 6000; 80% power to detect a 17% relative reduction in rate of OIs or death
Randomization: Permuted blocks, stratified by clinical site
Blinding: Unblinded
Statistical methods: Intention to treat analysis; Kaplan-Meier survival curves, Cox proportional hazards

Results
Participant flow: 5472 enrolled; 2720 in interrupted therapy (DC-drug) vs. 2752 in continuous therapy (VS) group. Primary end-point unknown in 32 from DC group, 41 from VS group. Mean follow-up 16mos.
Baseline data: No significant differences
Outcomes and estimation: Median duration of first period of interruption in DC group was 16.8mo. CD4 count 206 cells/mm3 less in DC vs. VS group. In DC vs. VS groups, OIs or death occurred in 120 (3.3 events per 100 person-years) vs. 47 participants, respectively (1.3 per 100 person-years) (HR 2.6, CI: 1.2-3.7, p< 0.001); major cardiovascular, renal or hepatic disease occurred in 65 vs. 39 participants, respectively (HR 1.7, CI: 1.1-2.5, p=0.009).
Ancillary analyses: HIV VL <400 for 28.8% vs. 72.3% of the time in DC vs. VS groups. No difference in grade 4 adverse events in DC vs. VS groups

Discussion
Conclusion: Interrupted ART, even when guided by CD4 counts, increased the risk of OIs and death compared to continuous treatment with ART and did not reduce the risk of adverse events.

Limitations: None identified

Funding: National Institute of Allergy and Infectious Diseases

---

Commentary   *Kemunto Mokaya, M.D., Resident in Internal Medicine*

SMART addressed the relative merits of continuous vs. CD4 count guided interrupted ART. With well-matched study groups at the start of the study, it showed no decrease in adverse events in patients receiving interrupted ART and actually showed increased risk of opportunistic infections and death when ART was interrupted at CD4 counts <250. On January 10, 2006, based on the data of harm in the interrupted treatment arm, the SMART trial was terminated. With the SMART study serving as a foundation, current guidelines reflect there is no evidence to recommend treatment interruptions of ART at lower CD4 counts (Cochrane Database 2006) and growing data that even at higher CD4 counts interrupted ART is still harmful [Antivir Ther. 2010;15 Suppl 1:17].

EFFECT OF EARLY VERSUS DEFERRED ANTIRETROVIRAL THERAPY FOR HIV ON SURVIVAL
Kitahata MM, Gange SJ, Abraham AG, et al. for the NA-ACCORD Investigators
New England Journal of Medicine 2009; 360:1815

Summary: Initiating antiretroviral therapy at CD4 counts between 350-500 or >500 reduces all-cause mortality in patients with asymptomatic HIV infection.

Introduction: When to initiate antiretroviral therapy (ART) in asymptomatic HIV+ patients has been controversial. At the time, WHO/CDC guidelines recommended initiation of ART at CD4 counts < 350 for asymptomatic patients with HIV. However, emerging data showed enhanced immunological function, better response to ART, and improved long term outcomes with early initiation of ART.

Objective: "To determine whether initiation of ART at early stages of HIV infection is associated with better survival rather than deferred therapy."

Methods
Trial Design: Retrospective cohort; two distinct cohorts from >60 centers in US and Canada
Participants: HIV+ patients; two parallel cohorts/analyses: patients with 1) CD4 350-500 and 2) CD4 >500; Excluded: no prior AIDS-defining illness, no previous ART
Interventions: Initiation of approved 3-drug ART at: 1) CD4 350-500 (early therapy) vs. CD 4 <350 (deferred therapy); 2) initiation of ART at CD4> 500 (early therapy) vs. CD4 <500 (deferred therapy)
Outcomes: Death from any cause
Sample size: CD4 350-500 cohort: 8,362 subjects totaling 23,977 person-years. CD4>500 cohort: 9,155 subjects totaling 26,439 person-years.
Randomization: None. Statistically "randomized" post-facto
Statistical methods: Wilcoxon, chi-squared test, Cox proportional hazards; inverse-probability weighting to approximate patient randomization

Results
Participant flow: CD4 350-500 cohort: 25% (2084) initiated ART within 6 mos, 75% (6278) deferred ART until CD4 <350. Of deferred therapy group, 55% (3449) dropped below CD4 <350 and 23% of these patients (803) started ART. CD4>500 cohort: 24% (9155) initiated ART, 42% (3881) dropped to CD4<500 and 14% (539) of these started ART. Patients not starting ART within 6mos were censored.
Baseline data: No significant differences
Outcomes and estimation: CD4 350-500 cohort: RR of death in deferred ART was 1.69 (CI 1.26-2.26, p <0.001); CD4>500 cohort: RR of death in deferred ART was 1.94 (CI 1.37-2.79, p <0.001). Cause of death available for only 16% of patients
Ancillary analyses: CD4 350-500 and >500 cohorts, increased risk of death with older age with deferred therapy. When IVDU and HCV excluded in both cohorts, RR death remained significantly increased with deferred ART. IVDU and HCV associated with overall higher risk of death
Harms: None identified

Discussion
Conclusion: Delaying ART in asymptomatic HIV+ patients until CD4 <350 and ≤500 is associated with an increase in all-cause mortality.
Limitations: Lack of randomization predisposes to selection bias; no measurement of adverse events or viral resistance associated with earlier ART; data censoring performed at 6mos

Funding: National Institutes of Health and Agency for Healthcare Research and Quality

---

Commentary   *Rachel Bender Ignacio MD, Resident in Internal Medicine*
When to start ART has been a rapidly moving target since 1996. The mortality benefit of initiating ART at CD4 cell count <200 has been well established by previous studies [NEJM 1997;337:725; Lancet 1998;351:543]. More recently, there has been compelling evidence from prospective cohorts that deferring combination therapy until a CD4 cell count of 251–350 is associated with higher rates of AIDS and death, suggesting that initiation of ART at a minimum CD4 350 is indicated [Lancet 2009;373:1352]. NA-ACCORD is one of the first trials to specifically address initiation of ART at CD4 cell counts >350. Strengths of the study include relatively large sample size, the primary end point of mortality, and minimization of lead-time bias by accessing data for patients prior to initiation of ART. Limitations include its retrospective design with potential selection bias of patients with "health seeking behavior" who chose to begin early ART. Data from patients not initiating ART within 6 months was censored. The authors also do not provide any data for measurement of adherence to ART in the early versus deferred therapy groups. Despite these caveats, NA-ACCORD adds to a growing body of literature supporting earlier initiation of ART. Ongoing RCTs evaluating early ART initiation include TEMPRANO (initiation of ART at CD > 350 vs. WHO guidelines in West Africa) and START (in recruitment phase).

TIMING OF INITIATION OF ANTIRETROVIRAL DRUGS DURING TUBERCULOSIS THERAPY (SAPIT)
Abdool Karim SS, Naidoo K, Grobler A, et al.
New England Journal of Medicine. 2010; 362: 697

Summary: In HIV + patients with CD4 counts <500 coinfected with tuberculosis, there is a survival benefit when anti-retroviral therapy is initiated concurrently with antitubercular therapy. There is increased risk of IRIS-related events but these events are non-fatal.

Introduction: In developing countries, tuberculosis (TB) is the most frequent cause of death in HIV infected patients. Despite WHO recommendations, anti-retroviral therapy is commonly delayed in the setting of active TB treatment due to risks of immune reconstitution inflammatory syndrome (IRIS), drug-drug interactions, side effects, and adherence.

Objective: "To determine the optimal time to initiate antiretroviral therapy in patients with HIV and tuberculosis coinfection who were receiving tuberculosis therapy."

Methods
Trial Design: Randomized, open-label, single center (outpatient clinic in S. Africa)
Participants: >18 years old; confirmed positive AFB smear and initiating standard TB treatment; confirmed HIV; CD4 <500; not on ART; Excluded: pregnancy, contraindication to therapy
Interventions: Adherence counseling, PCP prophylaxis, once daily didanosine, lamivudine, and efavirenz started within 4 weeks after: initiation/completion of intensive phase of TB therapy (early integrated) vs. completion of all phases of TB therapy (sequential therapy)
Outcomes: Primary: all-cause mortality, Secondary: toxicity, medication discontinuation, HIV RNA levels, TB outcomes, IRIS
Sample size: 642; 80% power to detect 60% mortality reduction
Randomization: Using sealed envelopes
Blinding: Unblinded
Statistical methods: Intention-to-treat analysis; Kaplan-Meier curves with log-rank test; proportional hazards regression

Results
Participant flow: 1331 individuals screened; 689 excluded; 642 patients enrolled and randomized (429 integrated therapy, 213 sequential therapy)
Baseline data: No significant differences
Outcomes and estimation: ART started approximately 70d vs. 260d after TB therapy initiated in integrated vs. sequential therapy group, respectively. Death rate of 5.4 vs. 12.1 per 100 person-years in integrated vs. sequential therapy group (CI 0.25-0.79, p=0.003). Decreased mortality in integrated therapy regardless of CD4 level
Ancillary analyses: Hazard ratio remained ~0.4 after adjustment for confounding factors (WHO HIV clinical stage, TB history, demographics). Similar ART adherence levels, TB outcomes, and non-IRIS adverse event rates between groups Proportion of patients with suppressed HIV RNA levels at 12 months was greater in integrated therapy group (90% vs. 77.8%, p=0.006).
Harms: IRIS diagnosed in 53 of 429 patients (12%) in integrated vs. 8 of 213 patients (4%) in sequential therapy groups (p<0.001), all IRIS events non-fatal

Discussion
Conclusion: Starting ART during rather than after TB therapy in HIV+ patients co-infected with TB yielded a 56% mortality reduction, attributable in part to a high death rate observed during the interval between completion of TB therapy and initiation of ART in the sequential therapy group.
Limitations: Causes of death surmised from non-standardized hospital charts. Extra-pulmonary and smear-negative TB excluded. High drop-out rate

Funding: PEPFAR, Global Fund, Comprehensive International Program of Research on AIDS

Commentary　　　　　　　　　　　　　*Emily A. Kendall, MD, Resident in Internal Medicine*
The SAPIT study was the first RCT to evaluate the mortality benefit to concomitant administration of ART in HIV/TB co-infected patients being treated for TB, showing a survival benefit to integrated HIV and TB therapy at CD4 counts <500. While there were more IRIS-related events in patients undergoing initiation of ART during treatment for TB, these events did not lead to mortality. Limitations include a large drop-out rate, lack of reporting of CD4 cell count at the initiation of ART and lack of generalizability due to inclusion of only smear-positive TB cases (a high proportion of HIV+ patients co-infected with TB are smear-negative). Concerns arose during the trial regarding the ethics of not immediately initiating ART in HIV/TB co-infected patients with CD4 cell count < 200 (WHO and S. African guidelines) and whether a trial was necessary given strong existing observational evidence for benefit with the initiation of ART during TB treatment. A subsequent trial (CAMELIA) demonstrated a mortality benefit to early ART in TB infected HIV+ patients with CD4 < 200 [NEJM. 2011; 365: 1471]

A Controlled Trial of Early Adjunctive Treatment with Corticosteroids for Pneumocystis Carinii Pneumonia in the Acquired Immunodeficiency Syndrome

Bozzette S, Sattler F, Chiu J, et al.
New England Journal of Medicine. 1990; 323: 1451

Summary: HIV+ patients with moderate to severe *Pneumocystis carinii* pneumonia have decreased rates of pulmonary failure and death with early adjunctive corticosteroid therapy.

Introduction: Adjunctive corticosteroid therapy may curb the extensive inflammatory lung damage associated with pneumocystis pneumonia (PCP) infection.

Objective: "To establish the improvement in clinical outcomes of adjunctive treatment with corticosteroids in patients with HIV infection and pneumocystis pneumonia, particularly given the concern that corticosteroids may result in exacerbation or development of opportunistic infections."

Methods
Trial Design: Randomized, multicenter (5 hospitals in California)
Participants: Adults with AIDS with presumed or confirmed PCP and < 36h of therapy. Excluded: age < 18, corticosteroid intolerance, mechanical ventilation, PaO2/FiO2 < 75
Interventions: Standard PCP therapy (TMP-SMX, pentamidine, or dapsone and TMP) vs. standard PCP therapy + corticosteroid (prednisone 40mg BID x 5d, 40mg QD x 5d, 20mg QD thereafter during duration of PCP therapy)
Outcomes: Primary: respiratory failure (death, mechanical ventilation, or PaO2/FiO2 < 75). Secondary: death, toxicity necessitating cessation of treatment
Sample size: 240; powered to detect 15% decrease in unfavorable outcome
Randomization: Centrally randomized
Blinding: Unblinded
Statistical methods: Chi-square, t-test, Mann-Whitney; Kaplan-Meier survival curves

Results
Participant flow: 333 enrolled, 82 excluded. Of remaining 251 patients, 225 had confirmed PCP and 26 classified as presumed PC
Outcomes and estimation: Majority of deaths and respiratory failure occurred in first 4 days. In steroid vs. standard groups, respectively, day 21 risk of respiratory failure 0.13 vs. 0.28 (p = 0.004); risk of death 0.09 vs. 0.18 (p=0.024); day 31 risk of respiratory failure 0.14 vs. 0.3 (p=0.004); risk of death 0.11 vs. 0.23 (p=0.009); day 81 risk of death 0.16 vs. 0.26 (p=0.026)
Ancillary analyses: Significantly decreased respiratory failure and death in moderate (PaO2/FiO2 250-350) and severe (PaO2/FiO2 75-250) strata in corticosteroid group. Greater change in PaO2/FiO2 ratio in corticosteroid group over duration of study. Benefit to adjunctive corticosteroid therapy maintained irrespective of center, type of PCP therapy. No difference in relapses between groups. Median duration of PCP therapy greater in corticosteroid vs. standard therapy groups (21 vs. 14d, p=0.002). Lower PaO2/Fi02 ratio was an independent predictor of respiratory failure.
Harms: Excess of localized herpetic lesions at day 84 in corticosteroid therapy group (26% vs. 15%, p=0.04, NNH=9)

Discussion
Conclusion: Early adjunctive corticosteroid therapy improves survival and lung function in AIDS patients with at least moderate PCP and has few adverse effects.
Limitations: Unblinded trial subject to bias. Corticosteroid group received longer treatment
Funding: California University-Wide AIDS Research Program

Commentary   *Allen Chang, MD, Resident in Internal Medicine*
This study showed that early initiation of corticosteroids in addition to standard PCP treatment decreased risk of respiratory failure and death at up to 84 days. These clinical benefits were most marked in patients with moderate to severe PCP pneumonia, a finding which was supported by a sister article in NEJM by Gagnon et al. Initiation of adjunctive corticosteroids did not significantly increase the incidence of common opportunistic infections other than localized herpetic lesions. Limitations of this study include lack of generalizability; the majority of patients included were young homosexual males with AIDS, owing in large part to the time the study was conducted (late 1980s). Confounding these results is the data that patients in the corticosteroid therapy group on average received a longer duration of PCP therapy. The 2004 IDSA guidelines support these findings, with severe PCP in HIV, defined by PaO2 < 70mmHg or A-a gradient of ≥ 35mmHg, warranting corticosteroid therapy as early as possible or within 72 hrs of initiating PCP therapy.

COMPARISON OF 8 VS. 15 DAYS OF ANTIBIOTIC THERAPY FOR VENTILATOR-ASSOCIATED PNEUMONIA IN ADULTS
Chastre J, Wolff M, Fagon J, et al.
Journal of the American Medical Association. 2003; 290:2588

Summary: Fifteen days of antimicrobial treatment for ventilator-associated pneumonia offered no benefit over 8 days of treatment in a selected ICU population.

Introduction: Nosocomial pneumonia is a frequent problem. However, randomized clinical trials assessing treatment duration are lacking.

Objective: "To determine whether 8 days is as effective as 15 days of antibiotic treatment of patients with microbiologically proven ventilator acquired pneumonia (VAP)."

Methods
Trial Design: Randomized, multi-center (51 ICUs in France)
Participants: Intubated (>48 hours) ICU patients with clinical suspicion of VAP, positive quantitative cultures of specimens obtained via bronchoscopy, and initiation of appropriate empiric antiobiotics within 24 hours (as determined by culture susceptibilities). Excluded: age <18; pregnant; little chance of survival with Simplified Acute Physiology Score (SAPS2) >65; neutropenia, AIDS, immunosuppression or long-term corticosteroids; concomitant extrapulmonary infection requiring prolonged anti-microbials
Interventions: 8 vs 15 days of clinician-selected antibiotic therapy
Outcomes: Primary: at 28 days: all cause death, pulmonary infection recurrence, and antibiotic-free days. Multiple secondary outcomes not discussed here
Sample size: 402; 90% power to detect 10% difference for mortality and reinfection (non-inferiority), and 20% difference for anti-biotic-free days (superiority)
Randomization: Central randomization using an interactive voice system performed day 3 post-bronchoscopy (to verify bacterial burden & appropriate initial antibiotic coverage)
Blinding: Double-blinded until day 8
Statistical methods: Intention-to-treat analysis; repeated 1-sided 90% CIs , nonparametric Wilcoxon test

Results
Participant flow: 1171 assessed. 386 deemed ineligible on day 1 and 383 deemed ineligible on day 3. 402 subjects randomized. Twenty-eight day follow-up
Baseline data: 9% more men in 8-day regimen (p=.046)
Outcomes and estimation: No difference in mortality or pulmonary infection recurrence rates. Patients in the 8-day regimen had more antibiotic-free days (p<.001). There were no differences in secondary outcomes.
Ancillary analyses: Logistic regression analyses did not substantially modify any of the outcomes. For primary infections caused by non-fermenting Gram-negative bacilli, a higher percentage of patients developed a significant recurrence in the 8-day group compared to the 15-day group (40.6% vs. 25.4%).
Harms: None identified

Discussion
Conclusion: There is no benefit associated with 15 instead of 8 days of antibiotics for VAP, and significantly greater antibiotic free-days with the 8-day regimen. Slightly fewer patients in the 15-day group had reinfection with non-fermenting Gram-negative bacilli. However the mortality and unfavorable outcomes did not differ even with these reinfections.
Limitations: The study could only be blinded through the first 8 days. The rigorous exclusion criteria eliminated 65% of ICU patients, limiting generalizability.

Funding: Research grant from the Délégation à la Recherche Clinique, Assistance Publique-Hopitaux de Paris

---

Commentary   *Renee Rutledge, MD, Resident in Internal Medicine*
This careful, well-designed study used strict definitions, obtained microbiologic diagnosis via bronchoscopy, and was blinded as long as clinically possible. It is often cited when withdrawing antibiotics in patients with nosocomial pneumonia of any kind, as the previous empiric recommendation was for 14-21 days of treatment for VAP. However, there are limitations to the generalizability, given that nearly 65% of ICU patients assessed were excluded. Based on the increased recurrence of pneumonia caused by non-fermenting gram-negative bacilli in the 8-day group, clinicians may consider 15 days of antimicrobial therapy in that specific patient population.

DEXAMETHASONE IN ADULTS WITH BACTERIAL MENINGITIS

De Gans J and Van De Beek D for the European Dexamethasone in Adulthood Bacterial Meningitis Study Investigators
New England Journal of Medicine. 2002; 347:1549

Summary: Early adjunctive treatment with dexamethasone improves both morbidity and mortality in adults with acute pneumococcal bacterial meningitis.

Introduction: Acute bacterial meningitis is associated with significant neurological morbidity in adults. Studies in animals have shown that adjuvant treatment with corticosteroids reduces these effects.

Objective: "To determine whether adjunctive dexamethasone treatment improves outcome in… patients [with acute pneumococcal bacterial meningitis]."

Methods

Trial Design: Randomized, multicenter (Europe)
Participants: Adults with suspected meningitis (defined by cloudy CSF, + gram stain, or CSF WBC>1000/mm³). Excluded: allergy to beta-lactam antibiotics or steroids; pregnancy; presence of a CSF shunt; previous antibiotics within last 48hrs; history of active TB or fungal infection; recent head trauma, neurosurgery, or PUD
Interventions: Dexamethasone 10mg IV Q6hrs x 4 days + Amoxicillin 2Gm IV Q4hrs x 7-10 days vs. Placebo + Amoxicillin 2Gm IV Q4hrs x 7-10 days. Dexamethasone or placebo administered 15-20 minutes prior to antibiotic administration.
Outcomes: Primary: Glasgow Outcome Score (GOS, neurological function score; favorable >5, unfavorable 1-4) at 8 weeks; Secondary: mortality or focal neurological deficits
Sample size: 300; 80% power to detect a 15% difference in GOS
Randomization: Concealed from investigators; computer generated at each hospital
Blinding: Double-blinded
Statistical methods: Intention-to-treat analysis; Student's t-test and Mann-Whitney U-test

Results

Participant flow: 301 enrolled and used for intention-to-treat analysis (157 to dexamethasone arm, 144 to placebo arm). 22 patients withdrew early (11 from each arm), resulting in 279 patients. At 8 weeks, 7 patients were lost to follow up. GOS performed on 262 patients
Baseline data: More patients with seizures in dexamethasone arm
Outcomes and estimation: Unfavorable GOS developed in 25% of controls vs. 15% of the dexamethasone arm (p = 0.03), a difference that remained after risk factor adjustment. Death by 8 weeks occurred in 15% of controls vs. 7% of the dexamethasone arm (p = 0.04, NNT=12). No significant difference in the development of focal neurological deficits
Ancillary analyses: Largest benefit seen in patients with moderate-to-severe neurological dysfunction. Patients with *S. pneumoniae* meningitis in dexamethasone arm had significant reduction in unfavorable neurological outcomes as compared to those in the placebo arm (p = 0.006), while those with other forms of bacterial meningitis did not.
Harms: None identified

Discussion

Conclusion: Early adjunctive treatment with dexamethasone improves both morbidity and mortality in adults with pneumococcal meningitis.
Limitations: None cited

Funding: Grant from NV Organon

Commentary   *Sarah Turbett, MD, Resident in Internal Medicine*
Over a decade old, this is still a fundamental study supporting the treatment of pneumococcal meningitis with dexamethasone. Since its publication, numerous studies have replicated the above findings. Most recently, a meta-analysis of more than 4000 patients found that adjuvant treatment with steroids resulted in a significant decrease in mortality in patients with pneumococcal meningitis and moderate to severe neurological dysfunction (RR 0.84, [0.72-0.98] and supports the use of this treatment in this patient population [Cochrane Database Syst Rev. 2010;9:CD004405]. Recent guidelines from Infectious Disease Society of America (IDSA), however, recommend adjunctive dexamethasone (0.15mg/kg Q6H x 2-4 days) with the first dose administered either 15-20 minutes prior or concomitant with the first dose of antibiotics in all patients with suspected pneumococcal meningitis regardless of neurological status in order to avoid delays in appropriate therapy [Clin Inf Dis 2004; 39: 1267].

ROLE OF ECHOCARDIOGRAPHY IN EVALUATION OF PATIENTS WITH STAPHYLOCOCCUS AUREUS
BACTEREMIA: EXPERIENCE IN 103 PATIENTS
Fowler, V, Li, J, Ryan, T et al.
Journal of the American College of Cardiology. 1997; 30:1072

Summary: Transesophageal echocardiography is more sensitive than transthoracic echocardiography in identifying signs of infective endocarditis in patients with *Staphylococcus aureus* bacteremia.

Introduction: The utility of transesophageal echocardiography (TEE) as compared to transthoracic echocardiography (TTE) in the diagnosis of infective endocarditis (IE) in patients with *Staphylococcus aureus* bacteremia (SAB) is unknown.

Objective: "To determine if TEE is diagnostically and prognostically useful in patients with SAB and to determine the relative diagnostic value of TTE and TEE compared with clinical variables for detecting IE in patients with SAB."

Methods
Trial Design: Prospective study, single center (Duke University Medical Center)
Participants: Hospitalized patients with ≥ 1 positive blood cultures for *S. aureus* and clinical signs of infection. Excluded: Age ≤ 18; polymicrobial infection; neutropenia; death prior to blood culture positivity; outpatient status
Clinical diagnosis of IE: Duke Criteria
-Definite IE: 2 major criteria; 1 major + 2 minor; or 5 minor criteria
Echocardiographic diagnosis of IE: Presence of vegetations, abscesses, paravalvular prosthetic valve regurgitation, new valvular regurgitation, or unexplained valve dysfunction
Interventions: TTE and TEE performed within 9 days of study entry
Outcomes: Findings suggestive of endocarditis on either TTE or TEE. Status of SAB at 12 weeks
Sample size: 103
Blinding: Echocardiographers were not blinded to clinical status. TEE performed after TTE but TEE's later re-interpreted in blinded manner. 20 randomly selected TEE's included in study to prevent bias created by knowing all patients had suspected SAB.
Statistical methods: Chi-squared test

Results
Participant flow: 284 potential patients. 109 dropped based on exclusion criteria. Of the 176 remaining eligible patients, 72 did not undergo TEE secondary to patient or physician refusal and 1 patient excluded as TTE was not performed. 103 patients remained for analysis.
Baseline data: No significant differences between patients with and without IE.
Outcomes and estimation: 26/103 of subjects met Duke criteria for definite IE. TEE had a higher sensitivity for detecting vegetations compared with TTE (100% vs. 32%, p = 0.004), driven by TEE's increased ability to detect small vegetations and abscesses. Specificity was similar between the two groups (TTE 100% vs. TEE 99%). TEE detected IE in 19% of patients with a negative TTE.
Ancillary analyses: No difference in cure rates of SAB between the two groups. None of the patients in whom IE was excluded based on Duke Criteria and negative TEE developed IE. Death due to sepsis was significantly more likely, however, in patients with IE (15% vs. 3%, p = 0.03).

Discussion
Conclusion: TEE has increased sensitivity as compared to TTE in the diagnosis of IE in patients with SAB.
Limitations: Only 59% eligible adult inpatients with SAB had TTE and TEE. Echocardiographers were not blinded. Sampling bias was possible, as physicians referred patients with higher suspicion for ECHO. The diagnosis of definite IE was made predominantly with ECHO and not pathology

Funding: N/A

Commentary   *Sarah Turbett, MD, Resident in Internal Medicine*
The role of TEE in the diagnosis of IE remains controversial. Based on the above study in *Staphylococcus aureus*, TEE is significantly more sensitive than TTE in diagnosing valvular vegetations. These findings have been supported by other studies, which have reported diagnostic sensitivities as low as 44% for TTE [J Am Coll Cardiol 1991; 18: 391]. Both the current ACC/AHA and IDSA guidelines recommend the use of TEE as the first diagnostic test in patients with moderate to high suspicion for IE or if TTE is unlikely to yield adequate imaging (e.g. COPD, morbid obesity) [Circulation 2005; 111: e394]. In addition, initial TEE has been shown to be a more cost effective test in the diagnosis of IE as compared to TTE [Am Jour Med 1999;107: 198].

EFFECTIVENESS OF PNEUMOCOCCAL POLYSACCHARIDE VACCINE IN OLDER ADULTS
Jackson LA, Neuzil KM, Onchee Y, et al.
New England Journal of Medicine. 2003; 348:1747

Summary: Pneumococcal polysaccharide vaccination is associated with reduced pneumococcal bacteremia but not community acquired pneumonia in adults greater than 65.

Introduction: In elderly patients, community-aquired pneumonia (CAP) is most commonly caused by *Streptococcus pneumoniae* infection. Prior studies evaluating pneumococcal polysaccharide vaccines have not shown consistent results but were underpowered.

Objective: "To evaluate the effectiveness of pneumococcal polysaccharide vaccine against community acquired pneumonia, as well as the more specific outcome of pneumococcal bacteremia."

Methods
Trial Design: Population-based retrospective cohort study, Washington state
Participants: HMO members ≥ 65 years of age and followed until death, disenrollment, or end of study
Intervention/Variable: Vaccination status
Outcomes: Primary: hospitalization for CAP, outpatient pneumonia, and pneumococcal bacteremia
Sample size: 47,365
Randomization: N/A
Blinding: N/A
Statistical methods: Crude event rates; multivariate Cox proportional-hazards model with time-varying covariates; models adjusted for age; sex; nursing-home residence; influenza vaccination; smoking status; diabetes mellitus, coronary artery disease, immunosuppression, chronic lung disease, dementia or stroke, and hospitalization for pneumonia and number of outpatient visits in year before study

Results
Participant flow: 47,365 persons were observed for 127,180 person-years. 26,313 persons were vaccinated prior to study, with an additional 10,869 vaccinated during the study period.
Baseline data: Compared with the unvaccinated group, the vaccinated group had more comorbidities, but fewer were nursing home residents.
Outcomes and estimation: 1428 patients hospitalized for CAP, 3061 patients with at least one episode of outpatient pneumonia, and 61 patients with pneumococcal bacteremia. After multivariate adjustment, vaccination was associated with 44% relative reduction in risk of pneumococcal bacteremia (p=0.03), but a higher risk of hospitalization with CAP. There was no association between vaccination and risk of outpatient pneumonia or death. Risk did not vary according to time since vaccination.
Ancillary analyses: Subgroup analysis in immunocompetent people found decreased risk of bacteremia (HR 0.46, p=0.02) and death (HR 0.88, p=0.005) from any cause in vaccinated group. There was no association in immunocompromised individuals.
Harms: None identified

Discussion
Conclusion: There is no evidence that pneumococcal polysaccharide vaccination is associated with a reduction in the risk of pneumonia from any cause. However, the vaccine is associated with reduced pneumococcal bacteremia and this supports its continued use.
Limitations: Observational study, limited by nonrandomized study and potential residual confounding. There was potential for misclassification bias.

Funding: Vaccine Safety Datalink contract with the American Association of Health Plans funded by the CDC

Commentary   *Vernon A. Rayford, MD, PharmD, Resident in Internal Medicine and Pediatrics*
Though an observational study, these results are applicable to the over 65 population and have implications for both inpatient and outpatient care. This study found that pneumococcal polysaccharide vaccination is associated with a reduced risk of pneumococcal bacteremia, but not outpatient pneumonia or hospitalization for community-acquired pneumonia. This lack of protection from outpatient pneumonia and the disparate finding of increased risk of hospitalization raise the question of whether conjugate pneumococcal vaccines should be used instead. A large, RCT of a 13-valent, expanded-serotype conjugate vaccine in older adults is underway and should provide further data [Neth J Med. 2008; 66: 378].

A Comparison of Vancomycin and Metronidazole for the Treatment of *Clostridium difficile*-Associated Diarrhea, Stratified by Disease Severity
Zar FA, Bakkanagari SR, Moorthi KM, Davis MB.
Clinical Infectious Diseases 2007; 45: 302

Summary: Oral vancomycin is superior to metronidazole for treatment of severe *C. difficile*-associated diarrhea, but equivalent for mild disease.

Introduction: *Clostridium difficile*-associated diarrhea (CDAD) is increasingly common and metronidazole treatment failure has been reported. No prior double-blinded RCTs have compared metronidazole to vancomycin therapy for CDAD.

Objective: To compare vancomycin treatment vs metronidazole treatment of CDAD, stratified by disease severity.

Methods
Trial Design: Randomized, single-center (Chicago)
Participants: Patients with diarrhea and either *C difficile* toxin A by stool assay or pseudomembranous colitis on endoscopy. Stratified by severity (mild vs. severe, defined as pseudomembranous colitis, ICU, or ≥2 of [age >60 yrs, temp >38.3°C, albumin <2.5 mg/dL, WBC >15,000]) Excluded: inability to take oral medications; life-threatening intraabdominal complications; prior treatment failure; pregnancy; allergy to study drug; treatment with study drug within 14 days
Interventions: Vancomycin liquid 125 mg PO QID + placebo tablet QID vs. metronidazole tablet 250 mg QID + placebo liquid QID x 10 days
Outcomes: Primary: cure (resolution of diarrhea by day 6 and negative *C difficile* toxin assay at days 6 and 10), treatment failure (persistence of diarrhea or positive *C difficile* assay after 6d, need for colectomy, or death after 5d), and relapse (recurrence of diarrhea and *C difficile* assay positive by day 21 after initial cure)
Sample size: 150; powered to detect 10% difference between treatment groups

Randomization: Card selected by pharmacy staff from sealed envelope
Blinding: Double-blinded
Statistical methods: As treated analysis; Fisher's exact test or unpaired *t* test

Results
Participant flow: 172 enrolled, 22 withdrew or died prior to completion of 10 days therapy, 150 completed protocol and were included in analysis. Twenty-one day follow-up
Baseline data: No significant differences
Outcomes and estimation: Cure in 84% in the metronidazole group and 97% in the vancomycin group (p=0.006). There was no difference in the rate of relapse after cure (14% metronidazole vs. 7% vancomycin, p=0.27).
Ancillary analyses: In patients with severe disease, cure occurred in 76% of the metronidazole group and 97% in the vancomycin group (p=0.02). In patients with mild disease, there was no difference in cure rate (metronidazole 90%, vancomycin 98%, p=0.36).
Harms: Rare nausea/vomiting, without differences between treatment groups

Discussion
Conclusion: Vancomycin is preferred over metronidazole for severe CDAD. There was no difference between the two agents for mild CDAD.
Limitations: As treated analysis. Vancomycin use may lead to increased vancomycin resistance, especially among enterococci.

Funding: Not declared

Commentary   *David A. Lyczkowski, MD, Resident in Internal Medicine and Pediatrics*
At the time this study was published, metronidazole was thought to be as effective as oral vancomycin for *Clostridium difficile*-associated diarrhea and was the first-line agent because of lower cost and concern for creating vancomycin-resistant enterococci. This RCT was the first to compare the two agents in a double-blinded, placebo-controlled fashion, and was the first to stratify according to disease severity (using a severity score developed for this study). The primary result, that cure rates with vancomycin were better than with metronidazole for severe disease, informed the latest IDSA/SHEA guideline, which states that oral vancomycin should be used as sole first-line agent for severe, uncomplicated disease. There is not yet consensus in the literature as to how severe disease is defined. However, guidelines still favor metronidazole for mild disease. Although this study did not employ intention-to-treat analysis and excluded from analysis 22 patients who had been randomized to treatment, including 8 who died within 5 days of initiation of treatment, it does not appear likely that the outcome was affected.

DEVELOPMENT OF AUTOANTIBODIES BEFORE THE CLINICAL ONSET OF SYSTEMIC LUPUS
ERYTHEMATOSUS
Arbuckle MR, McClain MT, Rubertone MV, et al.
New England Journal of Medicine. 2003; 349: 1526

Summary: The development of autoantibodies precedes the development of clinical systemic lupus erythematosus by months to years, depending on the type of antibody.

Introduction: Autoantibodies contribute to the pathogenesis of systemic lupus erythematosus (SLE); however, their natural history is unclear.

Objective: "To test the hypothesis that the appearance of autoantibodies precedes the diagnosis of SLE."

Methods
Trial Design: Retrospective case-control study
Participants: Military personnel with SLE (and matched controls) and serum samples before diagnosis of SLE
Data source: Prospectively collected serum and medical records from before and after the diagnosis of SLE
Outcomes: Time from first detection of autoantibodies at a ≥1:120 dilution to the onset of symptoms and diagnosis of SLE
Sample size: 130 cases, 260 controls
Statistical methods: Student's *t*-test, Kaplan-Meier product-limit curves

Results
Population: 64% women, 62% African-American; mean age at diagnosis was 30. Generally healthy apart from SLE

Outcomes: 115 (88%) of SLE patients had at least one positive antibody prior to diagnosis. Mean time to diagnosis from first positive ANA, antiphospholipid, anti-Ro, or anti-La Ab to diagnosis of SLE was 3.4 years. For anti-dsDNA it was 2.2 years and for anti-Sm and anti–nRNP it was 1.2 years. A similar trend was seen for time from antibody positivity to the first symptom of SLE. Antibodies were detected as early as 9 years before diagnosis.
Ancillary analyses: 3.8% of matched controls had positive antibodies (at a 1:120 dilution).

Discussion
Conclusion: Autoantibodies can be positive years before the first symptom of SLE. Anti-Sm and anti-nRNP may herald the diagnosis within months.
Limitations: For 69% of subjects, the first serum sample available was already positive for antibodies, hence possibly underestimating the time of antibody positivity to diagnosis. Military personnel may not be representative of the general population. Study did not address whether there is any utility in detecting the antibodies prior to diagnosis.

Funding: National Institutes of Health grants and the Department of Veterans Affairs

Commentary   *Laura Certain, MD, PhD Resident in Internal Medicine*
This study contributes to our understanding of the natural history of SLE, although it is unlikely to influence current practice. While the presence of ANA at ≥1:120, anti-Ro or La appears to increase the risk of SLE by at least a factor of 40, specific antibody testing in patients without symptoms of SLE is of little clinical benefit as there is no preventative treatment and the majority of the patients will not develop SLE. However, patients with positive antibodies - particularly anti-dsDNA, anti-nRNP and anti-Sm antibodies due to the proximity of their appearance in the blood and the onset of symptoms - should be monitored more closely for evidence of SLE.

CLINICAL AND RADIOGRAPHIC OUTCOMES OF FOUR DIFFERENT TREATMENT STRATEGIES IN
PATIENTS WITH EARLY RHEUMATOID ARTHRITIS (THE BeST STUDY)
Goekoop-Ruiterman YPM, de Vries-Bouwstra JK, Allaart CF, et al.
Arthritis and Rheumatism. 2005;52: 3381

Summary: Early and aggressive treatment of rheumatoid arthritis with combination therapy that includes prednisone or infliximab slows joint damage and improves functional status compared to single agent therapy.

Introduction: The optimal rheumatoid arthritis (RA) treatment strategy to reduce progression and improve function is not clear.

Objective: "What is the optimal therapeutic strategy in patients presenting with early rheumatoid arthritis to prevent long-term joint damage and functional decline?"

Methods
Trial Design: Randomized, multi-center (20 centers, Netherlands), open-label
Participants: Patients with early RA as defined by 1987 revised American College of Rheumatology (ACR) criteria. Excluded: contraindication to one of the study drugs
Interventions: Patients were randomized to:
1. Sequential monotherapy (15mg/week Methotrexate (MTX) titrated up followed by sulfasalazine (SSZ) monotherapy, leflunomide monotherapy, MTX with infliximab, gold with methylprednisolone, and then MTX with cyclosporine A (CSA) and prednisone);
2. Step-up combination therapy (15mg/week MTX titrated up followed by the addition of SSZ, hydroxychloroquine (HCQ), and then prednisone; if failure on all 4, switched to alternative regimen);
3. Initial combination therapy with tapered high-dose prednisone (7.5mg/week MTX, SSZ, and 60mg prednisone tapered over 7 wks; if improvement, prednisone was tapered off, then MTX was tapered off; if failure, MTX was augmented and then the combination was replaced with other combinations);
4. Initial combination therapy with infliximab (25-30mg/week MTX with 3mg/kg infliximab which was uptitrated if failure and ultimately switched to alternative regimen if no response; if improvement, infliximab was reduced);
Outcomes: Primary: functional ability measured by the Health Assessment Questionnaire (D-HAQ) and radiographic joint damage of hands/feet. Secondary: 20%, 50%, 70% improvement in ACR response criteria and clinical remission (DAS$_{44}$<1.6)
Sample size: 508; 80% power to assess a 0.2 difference in D-HAQ and a 20% change in the radiograph score

Statistical methods: Intention to treat analysis; one-way analysis of variance; Tukey's honestly significant difference test; Kruskal-Wallis test; Mann-Whitney U test; chi-square test

Results
Participant flow: 508 randomized (equal among groups). Equivalent amounts of patient dropout from each group. One-year follow-up
Baseline data: No significant differences
Outcomes: Improved DHAQ scores at 3mo with initial combination therapy with prednisone (group 3) or infliximab (group 4; D-HAQ=0.6 in both groups) compared to groups 1 and 2 (D-HAQ=1.0 in both groups; p<0.001). At 1 yr, the D-HAQ scores were 0.7 in groups 1 and 2 and 0.5 in groups 3 and 4 (p=0.009). Groups 3 and 4 had less progression of radiographic joint damage compared to groups 1 and 2 (p<0.001). ACR 20 and 70 were reached earlier by groups 3 and 4.
Harms: 41% of patients experienced ≥1 adverse effect (no difference among groups)

Discussion
Conclusion: Initial therapy with infliximab or prednisone in combination with disease-modifying anti-rheumatic drugs (DMARDs) accelerated functional improvement and curbed radiographic progression of joint damage compared with sequential monotherapy or step-up combination therapy with DMARDs alone.
Limitations: Patients not blinded. Initial MTX dose was different between the groups. No post-hoc analysis by severity of disease

Funding: Dutch College of Health Insurances, Centocor Inc. and Schering-Plough BV

Commentary   *Zachary S. Wallace, MD Resident in Internal Medicine*
Early RA is important to recognize and treat aggressively as longer active disease duration is associated with poor response to treatment. The BeSt study compared four treatment strategies, one of which (group 3) had previously been evaluated [Lancet. 1997;350;309]. This study demonstrated that compared to conventional treatment at the time (i.e. group 1) early combination therapy in RA was effective in preventing functional decline and radiographic progression at one year. Subsequent studies have demonstrated sustained effect at longer follow-up [Ann Intern Med. 2007;146:406; Arthritis Rheum. 2009;60:1222; Ann Rheum Dis. 2010 Jul;69(7):1298-304]. The ACR recommends different treatment strategies based on a patient's severity of disease, which the BeSt study did not examine [Arthritis Rheum. 2008;59(6):762-84].

DOES THIS PATIENT HAVE TEMPORAL ARTERITIS?
Smetana GW and Shmerling RH
Journal of the American Medical Association. 2002; 287: 92

Summary: Age >50, jaw claudication, diplopia, temporal artery abnormalities and ESR are valuable tools in the diagnosis of giant cell arteritis.

Introduction: Giant cell arteritis (GCA) is the most common primary vasculitis and can cause significant morbidity, most notably vision loss. However, GCA is frequently difficult to diagnose and a high level of suspicion is required.

Objective: "To determine the accuracy of historical features, physical examination, and erythrocyte sedimentation rate (ESR) in the diagnosis of temporal arteritis."

Methods
Trial Design: Systematic review
Studies Included: 21 studies (4 prospective and 17 retrospective) where at least 90% of study subjects underwent temporal artery (TA) biopsy.
Outcomes: Diagnostic value of historical, physical exam features and laboratory data in the diagnosis of GCA.
Sample size: 2680 patients from 21 studies.
Statistical methods: Likelihood ratios (LR), sensitivity and specificity. Summary measures obtained using a random effects measure.

Results
Baseline data: 2680 patients included, 1050 (39%) had positive temporal artery biopsy results.
Outcomes:
Historical Features: Jaw claudication (LR+ 4.2) and diplopia (LR+ 3.4) were found to be predictive of a positive TA biopsy. However both features had low sensitivity – 34% and 9% respectively. The most sensitive historical feature was age > 50 (99% sensitive). Notably LRs for fever, polymyalgia rheumatica, visual loss and temporal headache were not significant.

Physical Examination: Temporal artery abnormalities were shown to be the most useful physical exam feature. Enlarged, beaded or tender temporal arteries had a LR+ of 4.6, 4.3 and 2.6 respectively (combined 65% sensitivity). The presence of synovitis had a LR+ of 0.41, making the diagnosis of GCA less likely. Scalp tenderness was not a good predictor of GCA.

Laboratory Data: An abnormal ESR had a sensitivity of 96% (LR- 0.2), making it a useful feature to rule-out GCA. An ESR < 50mm/hr had a LR+ of 0.35 and an ESR > 100 conferred a LR+ of 1.9.

Discussion
Conclusion: A normal ESR and age < 50 make GCA unlikely. Jaw claudication, diplopia and temporal artery abnormalities increase the likelihood of GCA.

Limitations: Including only high-risk patients causes verification bias, which may underestimate the predictive value of findings. Predictive values of co-existing features which are typically present in GCA were not explored.

Commentary   *Eli Miloslavsky, MD, Resident in Internal Medicine*
GCA, the most common primary vasculitis, poses a significant challenge to the clinician given the broad array of historical and physical findings that may raise suspicion for the disease. This study adds to our understanding of the presenting features of GCA. However, no one feature is diagnostic of GCA and patients often have a constellation of findings which was not addressed in this study. While temporal artery biopsy is a useful diagnostic tool, biopsies have a false negative rate of at least 5-9% [Lancet. 1983;2:1217; Mayo Clin Proc. 2004;79:483]. Therefore, the history, physical examination and laboratory studies play an important role in the diagnosis of GCA. Studies suggest patients with suspected GCA should be started on glucocorticoid therapy before they undergo biopsy as this is unlikely to influence the diagnostic yield [Ann Intern Med. 1994; 120:987]. Bilateral biopsy may increase diagnostic yield as the biopsies can be discordant in up to 13% of cases [J Rheumatol. 2009;36(4):794].

INFLIXIMAB (CHIMERIC ANTI-TUMOR NECROSIS FACTOR α MONOCLONAL ANTIBODY) VERSUS PLACEBO IN RHEUMATOID ARTHRITIS PATIENTS RECEIVING CONCOMITANT METHOTREXATE: A RANDOMISED PHASE III TRIAL (ATTRACT)
Maini R, St Clair E, Breedveld F, et al. for the ATTRACT Study Group
Lancet. 1999; 354: 1932

Summary: Methotrexate combined with infliximab is safe and more effective than methotrexate monotherapy for treatment of recalcitrant rheumatoid arthritis.

Introduction: New therapies are needed for rheumatoid arthritis (RA) patients who don't tolerate, or respond poorly to, methotrexate (MTX).

Objective: "To determine whether infliximab, at two doses every 4 or 8 weeks, added to therapeutic doses of methotrexate, is safe and effective in relief of signs and symptoms of disease."

Methods
Trial Design: Randomized, multi-center (34 sites in U.S and Europe)
Participants: Patients with active RA (6 swollen joints and elevated inflammatory markers or AM stiffness) despite continuous MTX therapy (≥12.5 mg/wk) for at least 3mos. Excluded: confounding disease that would make RA activity difficult to track or uncontrolled systemic disease, disease-modifying anti-rheumatic drug (DMARD) besides MTX, IV/IM/IA corticosteroid in past month, serious infection within 3mo, any chronic infection, recent active TB or malignancy
Interventions: In addition to MTX (patients' baseline dose) all patients received infusions of either placebo or infliximab (INF) at weeks 0, 2 and 6. Patients were then randomized to: placebo infusions vs. one of four INF infusions (3mg/kg every 4wk or 6wk; 10mg/kg every 4wk or 6wk)
Outcomes: 20% improvement in RA by American College of Rheumatology (ACR) criteria* at week 30; Secondary: ACR 50% & 70% improvement
Sample size: 428; 90% power to detect a 45% difference in clinical response
Randomization: Randomized, stratified by site

Blinding: Double-blinded
Statistical methods: Intention-to-treat analysis; chi-squared test, ANOVA, Fisher's exact tests

Results
Participant flow: 428 randomized, 35 from placebo and 47 from the four INF groups withdrew. Thirty-week follow-up.
Baseline data: No significant differences between groups. 80% female, average disease duration 7-9 years, 80% - most failed 2+ DMARDS other than MTX in the past, over 50% receiving steroids.
Outcomes and estimation: More patients receiving any dose of INF achieved 20% ACR response (50% vs. 20%, p<0.001), ACR50 (25% vs. 5%, p<0.001) and ACR70 (8-18% vs. 0%, p<0.01). Improved disease activity and general health was observed in all INF groups.
Ancillary analyses: 3 mg/kg every 8 weeks (the lowest dose used) showed sustained response at 30wk with equivalent efficacy to 3 mg/kg every 4 weeks and 10 mg/kg every 4 or 8 weeks.
Harms: No increase in adverse events vs. placebo; one case of drug-induced lupus in INF group

Discussion
Conclusion: INF improves RA in ≥50% patients with disease uncontrolled by MTX alone; INF 3mg/kg every 8wk is equally effective as the other doses and frequencies studied.
Limitations: Short follow-up (30 weeks). Excluded patients with early RA

Funding: Centocor Inc., Malvern, PA [manufacturer of Remicade (infliximab)]

Commentary   *John Korman, MD, Resident in Internal Medicine*
The well-designed phase III ATTRACT trial demonstrated the relative safety and efficacy of infliximab in the management of chronic RA. It was one of the first anti-TNF trials in the treatment of RA and ushered in the biologics era of therapies targeting specific cytokines. Currently, anti-TNF agents are indicated for early aggressive disease or chronic disease not responsive to MTX although other treatment strategies are also effective [Arthritis Rheum. 2008;59:762]. The study did not address the treatment of early RA or the efficacy of anti-TNF monotherapy. It is notable that two subjects receiving infliximab died from infectious etiologies in the study's next 6 months. Subsequent meta-analysis confirmed the increased risk of serious infection and malignancy in RA patients receiving anti-TNF treatment [JAMA. 2006;295:2275]. It is recommended that all patients are screened for TB and those at high risk screened for HBV and HCV prior to the initiation of anti-TNFs [Ann Rheum Dis. 2010;69:i2-i29]. In the ATTACH study of infliximab for heart failure, NYHA Class III /IV patients experienced increased rates of hospitalization and death, making anti-TNFs contraindicated in such patients [Circulation. 2003;107:3133].

SAFETY AND EFFICACY OF LONG-TERM INTRAARTICULAR STEROID INJECTIONS IN OSTEOARTHRITIS OF
THE KNEE: A RANDOMIZED, DOUBLE-BLIND, PLACEBO-CONTROLLED TRIAL
Raynauld JP, Buckland-Wright C, Ward R, et al.
Arthritis Rheum. 2003; 48: 370

Summary: Long-term intraarticular steroid injections for treatment of osteoarthritis of the knee appear to be
safe but have limited efficacy at symptom reduction.

Introduction: Intraarticular (IA) steroid injections
are used in the management of pain relief in
osteoarthritis (OA) with little published data on
the long-term effects.

Objective: "To evaluate the safety and efficacy of
long-term intraarticular steroid injections for knee
pain related to osteoarthritis."

Methods
Trial Design: Randomized, outpatient
rheumatology clinics at single center (Montreal)
Participants: Adults (40-80 years old) with knee
OA (Kellgren/Lawrence grade 2-3 of 4) not
responsive to acetaminophen/NSAID treatment.
Excluded: Patients with chondrocalcinosis,
infection, isolated patellofemoral OA, secondary
OA, IA steroids in past 6mos, radiographic grade 4
OA, severe functional disability, contralateral total
knee replacement, candidate for immediate surgery
Interventions: IA triamcinolone acetonide (40mg)
vs. IA saline every three months for 2 years.
Patients evaluated before each injection
Outcomes: Primary: radiographic progression of
joint space narrowing of injected knee after 2 years
and pain subset of the WOMAC scale (a validated
index on pain/stiffness/function). Secondary:
Total WOMAC score, physician assessment,
patient's global assessment and pain assessment,
range of motion (ROM), 50-ft walking time
Sample size: 68; 80% power to detect 25%
decrease in progression of joint space narrowing at
2 years
Randomization: Concealed from investigators;
based on table of randomly assorted numbers
Blinding: Assessors blinded; injectors unblinded.
Statistical methods: Intention-to-treat and area
under the curve (AUC) analysis

Results
Participant flow: 68 randomized; 66 completed
trial. Two-year follow-up.
Baseline data: 66% had grade 2 of 4 OA; more
females in IA steroid group (74% vs. 61%)
Outcomes and estimation: No differences in
change in joint space width or pain score. Joint
space width was unchanged over course of study.
Pain score improved by ~25% in both groups. No
differences in secondary outcome measures at end
of study; of note, after 1 year, improved ROM in
IA steroid group (p=0.05), which did not persist at
2 years.
Ancillary analyses: AUC analysis showed
significantly less night pain and stiffness (p<0.05)
in IA steroid group.
Harms: No adverse events in either group.

Discussion
Conclusion: Long-term IA steroid injections of
the knee appear to be safe but have limited
efficacy at symptom reduction. There is an
improvement in night pain and stiffness.

Limitations: New publications during the study
demonstrated that the study was insufficiently
powered both for radiographic and clinical
measures of disease; no wash-out period for
NSAIDs or analgesics; 3 month evaluations may
have missed short term improvement from steroid
injections.

Funding: Fonds de la Recherche en Santé du
Québec

Commentary   *Annie Lee, MD, Resident in Internal Medicine*
While underpowered, this was the first study to demonstrate long-term safety of IA steroids for treatment
of OA of the knee. The lack of significant long-term efficacy demonstrated by this study has since been
supported by several meta-analyses. However, IA steroids have been found to be effective for short term
pain relief for up to 4 to 24 weeks [BMJ. 2004;328:869; Cochrane Database Syst Rev. 2006:CD005328; Eur J Pain
2007;11:125]. IA steroid injections are recommended by the ACR for patients with moderate to severe pain
not responsive to NSAIDs or acetaminophen and for patients with significant signs of inflammation [ACR
guidelines, http://www.rheumatology.org/practice/clinical/guidelines/oa-mgmt.asp]. IA steroid therapy is one component
of OA treatment which includes weight reduction, physical therapy, knee bracing, footwear modification,
thermal therapy, acupuncture, acetaminophen, oral and topical NSAIDs, glucosamine chondroitin, IA
hyaluronate injections and total knee replacement [Osteoarthritis Cartilage 2008;16:137].

COMPARISON OF AN ANTI-INFLAMMATORY DOSE OF IBUPROFEN, AN ANALGESIC DOSE OF IBUPROFEN, AND ACETAMINOPHEN IN THE TREATMENT OF PATIENTS WITH OSTEOARTHRITIS OF THE KNEE
Bradley JD, Brandt KD, Katz BP, et al.
New England Journal of Medicine. 1991; 325: 87

Summary: Acetaminophen, ibuprofen at antiinflammatory doses, and ibuprofen at analgesic doses were equally effective in short-term treatment of knee osteoarthritis.

Introduction: Joint pain from osteoarthritis (OA) is often treated with non-steroidal anti-inflammatory drugs (NSAIDs), but their comparative effectiveness is unknown.

Objective: "In this study we compare a pure analgesic, acetaminophen, with an NSAID, ibuprofen, in short-term, symptomatic treatment of osteoarthritis of the knee."

Methods
Trial Design: Randomized, single center (Indiana)
Participants: ≥30years old with knee pain, radiographic evidence of mild to moderate osteoarthritis, ambulatory without assist devices. Excluded: patients with concomitant disease causing lower extremity pain and those with contraindications to study medications.
Interventions: Daily 4000mg acetaminophen vs. 1200mg ibuprofen (analgesic dose) vs. 2400mg ibuprofen (anti-inflammatory dose)
Outcomes: Primary/secondary not specified. (1) Disability scores on Stanford Health Assessment Questionnaire (2) Rest pain score (3) Walking pain score (4) Time needed to walk 50ft (5) Physician's assessment of disease
Sample size: 204; 90% power to detect changes >20% in visual-analogue pain scores and >10% in disability
Randomization: Details not specified, concealed from investigators
Blinding: Double-blinded
Statistical methods: Intention-to-treat analysis; paired t-tests or chi-square test; multivariate analysis

Results
Participant flow: 244 recruited, 204 enrolled, 195 randomized, 11 lost to follow-up (5 in acetaminophen group, 3 in low-dose ibuprofen, 3 assigned in high-dose ibuprofen) and 144 completed trial. Four-week follow-up
Baseline data: 75% female, 40% with moderate to severe disease according to physician assessment. No significant differences between groups
Outcomes and estimation: All 3 groups had a 2-15% improvement in all outcome measures which did not reach statistical significance, with the exception of rest pain, which decreased more in both ibuprofen groups vs. acetaminophen (p=0.05).
Ancillary analyses: Comparable compliance of 88% in all 3 groups
Harms: GI system most often affected. Trend toward increase in nausea and dyspepsia in high dose ibuprofen

Discussion
Conclusion: High dose ibuprofen was not superior to low dose ibuprofen or acetaminophen in pain relief or functional improvement; all groups had symptomatic relief over the month-long study period.
Limitations: Short, 4-week treatment follow-up; only assessed mild-moderate OA of the knee.

Funding: National Institute of Arthritis and Musculoskeletal and Skin Diseases

---

Commentary   *Annie Lee, MD, Resident in Internal Medicine*
OA affects over 30% of patients greater than 70 years of age and is the world's 4th leading non-fatal health burden [Ann Intern Med 2011;154:217]. In addition to nonpharmacologic treatment (weight reduction, physical therapy, knee bracing, use of cane, footwear modification, thermal therapy, acupuncture), pharmacologic treatment is often added for pain relief and functional improvement in OA of the knee. This study's finding of comparable responses to acetaminophen vs. NSAIDs in mild-to-moderate OA joint pain was borne out in subsequent studies [Arthritis Rheum 1993;36:1196; Semin Arthritis Rheum 1997;27:755]. However, several meta-analyses found superiority of ibuprofen vs. acetaminophen [Ann Rheum Dis 2004 63:901; Cochrane Database Syst Rev 2006:CD004257]. In deciding on pharmacologic treatment for knee OA, consideration should be given to the patient's comorbidities, including risk of GI bleed and kidney injury.

THE 1982 REVISED CRITERIA FOR THE CLASSIFICATION OF SYSTEMIC LUPUS ERYTHEMATOSUS
Tan EM, Cohen AS, Fries JF, et al.
Arthritis and Rheumatism.1982;25:1271

Summary: For the purposes of research and to assist physicians in the clinical setting, 11 criteria were found to be sensitive and specific for the diagnosis of systemic lupus erythematous when at least 4 of 11 are fulfilled by a patient.

Introduction: The ability to detect anti-dsDNA, ANA and serum complement prompted a revision of the diagnostic criteria published in 1971.

Objective: "The 1971 criteria [...] were revised and updated to incorporate new immunologic knowledge and improve disease classification."

Methods

Trial Design: An expert committee chose 30 potential criteria (including the 1971 criteria) and compared the presence of these criteria in SLE patients to matched controls.

Participants: 18 investigators from "major clinics" were asked to submit data on 10 SLE and 10 matched patients (for age, sex, and race) with other connective tissue diseases (e.g., RA, scleroderma, dermatomyositis, etc). Patients from the Scleroderma Criteria Cooperative Study (SCCS) database were used for criteria validation.

Intervention: 30 clinical variables were compared in SLE and control patients.

Outcomes: Specificity and sensitivity of each variable as well as combinations of variables for the diagnosis of SLE

Sample size:
Derivation cohort: 117 SLE patients and 108 matched controls
Validation cohort: 60 SLE and 54 controls
Second validation cohort: 172 SLE, 299 scleroderma and 119 dermatomyositis patients from the SCCS database.

Statistical methods: Multivariate analysis, cluster analysis, chi-square test

Results

Baseline data: The control population was matched for age, sex, and race to SLE patients.

Outcomes and estimation: 11 criteria were chosen with an overall sensitivity and specificity of 96% for the diagnosis of SLE in the validation cohort when 4 of 11 criteria were fulfilled. The most sensitive variables included were ANA [99% (LR- 0.02)] and arthritis [86% (LR- 0.38)], although neither was specific [49% (LR+ 1.9) and 37% (LR+ 1.4) respectively]. Anti-DNA and anti-Smith were highly specific with a specificity of 95% and 92%, respectively. Each of the other variables included in the criteria were over 85% specific (sensitivity 12-57%).

Ancillary analyses: The criteria were 83% sensitive and 89% specific when tested against the second validation cohort from the SCCS data.

Discussion

Conclusion: Overall, there was significant continuity between the 1971 and 1982 criteria (16 criteria of the original 21 remained). Adding ANA improved sensitivity. Including anti-DNA and anti-Smith improved the specificity of the criteria. Alopecia and Reynaud's, present in the 1971 criteria, were excluded in the 1982 criteria.

Limitations: SLE patients in the derivation and the first validation cohort were picked by investigators, limiting generalizability. Hence, the criteria did not perform as well when tested against the SCCS data. Some of the patients in the SCCS database did not have data available regarding the presence of anti-DNA and anti-Smith autoantibodies.

Commentary   *Zachary S. Wallace, MD Resident in Internal Medicine*
The inclusion of ANA positivity in the revised 1982 criteria improved the ability to identify SLE patients with high sensitivity and specificity. However, a key goal of creating such criteria was to select patients for inclusion in clinical trials. Therefore, the 1982 criteria must be employed with caution when used in the clinical diagnosis of SLE. The most important limitation is that patients with limited or atypical forms of the disease were excluded, as evidenced by only 83% sensitivity when tested against the SCCS database. Furthermore, since SLE clinical trials require the fulfillment of the 1982 criteria, the generalizability of such studies may be further limited [J Rheumatol. 2002;29:2545]. Since the introduction of these diagnostic criteria, the immunologic disorder criterion has been broadened to include the presence of lupus anticoagulant and IgG or IgM anti-cardiolipin [Arthritis Rheum. 1997;40:1725]. In an effort to improve diagnostic relevance, an expert group (Systemic Lupus International Collaborating Clinics -- SLICC) derived and tested a new set of criteria on a cohort of patients considered to have SLE based on a thirty-two person panel starting in 2003. In patients who have 4 criteria from this revised list, at least one clinical and one immunologic (or biopsy proven lupus nephritis with +ANA or dsDNA), there is improved sensitivity but not specificty for detecting clinical disease. [Arthritis Rheum 2012; 64: 2677]

A MULTICENTER RANDOMIZED CONTROLLED CLINICAL TRIAL OF TRANSFUSION REQUIREMENTS IN CRITICAL CARE
Hébert P, Wells G, Blajchman M, et al. for the TRICC Group
New England Journal of Medicine. 1999; 340: 409

Summary: In critically ill patients who do not have active blood loss or ischemia, a transfusion threshold of Hg 7 g/dL is equivalent (and possibly superior) to a transfusion threshold of Hg 10 g/dL.

Introduction: Anemia and tissue hypoxia are common in the critical care setting. Although the transfusion of red blood cells (RBC) can improve oxygen delivery, there are also deleterious consequences (volume overload, infection, others). The break-even point for the benefit of transfusion in critical care patients who are neither ischemic nor hemorrhaging, had not been established.

Objective: "To determine whether a restrictive approach to red cell transfusion that maintains Hg between 7-9 g/dL is equivalent to a more liberal strategy of maintaining Hg between 10-12 g/dL in critically ill patients."

Methods
Trial Design: Randomized, multi-center (25 ICUs in Canada), non-inferiority study
Participants: Euvolemic adult ICU patients with Hg ≤ 9 g/dL within the first 72hrs of the ICU admission and expected ICU length of stay (LOS) >24 hrs. Excluded: chronic anemia, active blood loss, pregnancy or expected imminent death
Interventions: Randomized to goal Hgb of either >7 g/dL or > 10 g/dL
Outcomes: Primary: death at 30d Secondary: death during ICU stay, hospitalization, or at 60d; number of organs failed, ICU length of stay (LOS), hospital LOS
Sample size: 838; powered to detect an absolute difference in the 30d mortality rate of 5.5 percent
Blinding: Unblinded
Statistical methods: Intention to treat analysis; ANOVA, Fisher's exact test, Kaplan-Meier survival curves, independent t-test, chi-square test

Results
Participant flow: 6451 assessed; 2039 screened for consent; 838 consented and randomized, 9 withdrew (4 from liberal transfusion strategy, 5 from restrictive)
Baseline data: Similar age, APACHE score, and other disclosed variables including "cardiovascular disease," but ACS and CAD not explicitly stated
Outcomes: Rate of death at 30d was equivalent between groups. There was also no difference in in-hospital/60-day mortality, LOS, or organ dysfunction.
Ancillary analyses: In analysis restricted to younger patients (<55 y/o) or those with APACHE score <20 (less acutely ill), there was increased mortality in the liberal transfusion strategy (Hg > 10 g/dL) (p=0.02 for both). MIs, pulmonary edema, angina, ARDS were also significantly more frequent in the liberal transfusion group.

Discussion
Conclusion: A goal Hg of 7 g/dL is at least as effective as, and possibly superior to, a goal Hg of 10 g/dl in critically ill patients who are not actively bleeding or ischemic.
Limitations: Patients with severe cardiac disease were disproportionately not included due to refusal to enroll by the attending physician. Treatment arms were not blinded and may have influenced use of other interventions.

Funding: Medical Research Council of Canada, Bayer

Commentary   *Jonathan Peled, M.D., Ph.D, Resident in Internal Medicine*
The TRICC trial offers the best available data for the management of subacute anemia in the absence of active blood loss or ischemia. Although lower transfusion thresholds have not been as rigorously evaluated, smaller trials have shown increased mortality that begins once the hemoglobin is allowed to decrease below 7g/dL [Transfusion 2002;42:812]. It should be emphasized that this transfusion threshold is not applicable to patients with active blood loss, those with chronic anemia prior to onset of critical illness or to patients with active ischemia (e.g. rising lactic acidosis or acute coronary syndrome), as these groups were largely excluded in this trial. In addition to setting practice standards for the use of RBC transfusion in critically ill patients, this emphasizes the morbidity (e.g. fluid overload, infection, TRALI) and mortality associated with liberal transfusions. Subsequent retrospective analyses have further demonstrated that RBC transfusion is an independent predictor of organ dysfunction and mortality [JAMA 2002;288:1499; Crit Care Med 2004;32:39].

LOW-MOLECULAR-WEIGHT HEPARIN VERSUS A COUMARIN FOR THE PREVENTION OF RECURRENT
THROMBOEMBOLISM IN PATIENTS WITH CANCER (CLOT)
Lee A, Levine M, Baker R, et al. for the CLOT Investigators
New England Journal of Medicine. 2003;349: 146

Summary: Low-molecular-weight heparin decreases the risk of recurrent venous thromboembolism as compared to oral vitamin K antagonists in patients with malignancy.

Introduction: Cancer patients treated with oral vitamin K antagonists for venous thromboembolism (VTE) have higher rates of recurrent thrombosis and bleeding than patients without active malignancy.

Objective: "We compared the efficacy of a low-molecular-weight heparin with that of an oral anticoagulant agent in preventing recurrent thrombosis in patients with cancer."

Methods
Trial Design: Randomized, multicenter (Canada, USA, Europe, New Zealand/Australia)
Participants: 676 adult patients with active cancer and documented proximal VTE or PE. Excluded: < 40kg, ECOG performance status 3 or 4, received heparin product at therapeutic dose for > 48 hrs, bleeding within 2 weeks, renal insufficiency, or heparin contraindicated (e.g. HIT)
Interventions: Dalteparin (200 IU/kg daily x 1 month followed by 150 IU/kg daily x 5 months) or coumarin derivative (coumadin in all centers except Spain/Netherlands) with target INR 2.5
Outcomes: Recurrence of symptomatic VTE within 6 months. Secondary: rates of bleeding, major bleeding and mortality
Sample size: 676; powered to detect 50% reduction in primary outcome
Randomization: Randomized by clinical center
Blinding: Open label for patients and investigators; blinded adjudication committee reviewed all events
Statistical methods: Intention to treat analysis; Kaplan-Meier method, two-sided log rank test

Results
Participant flow: 1303 enrolled; 676 randomized (439 excluded and 188 did not sign consent); 50% allocated to each treatment group; 672 completed protocol (4 excluded for lack of initial VTE)
Baseline data: No significant differences
Outcomes and estimation: Dalteparin reduced the probability of recurrent VTE, 9% vs. 17% in the oral anticoagulant arm (HR 0.48; P=0.002)
Ancillary analyses: There was no difference in mortality (p=.53) between the treatment groups with 90% of deaths occurring secondary to cancer progression (39% in dalteparin group vs. 41% in vitamin K antagonist group). In the oral anticoagulant subgroup, INRs were therapeutic 46% of the time (38% of thrombotic events in this group occurred with INR<2.0; 50% of major bleeding occurred with INR>3).
Harms: No significant difference in rates of major bleeding (p=.27) or any bleeding (p=.09).

Discussion
Conclusion: Dalteparin was superior to vitamin k antagonists in preventing recurrent VTE with no excessive bleeding risk in patients with active malignancy.
Limitations: Open-label design, higher cost for low-molecular-weight heparin (LMWH), self-injection feasibility, and unclear optimal dosing of LMWH at the time of the trial.

Funding: Pharmacia (makers of Dalteparin)

Commentary   *David Sallman, MD, Resident in Internal Medicine*
The CLOT trial demonstrated that the risk of recurrent VTE in cancer patients could be reduced by the use of LMWH as compared to oral vitamin K antagonists without increased bleeding. Although the trial was an open label study, attempts were made to limit bias through blinded adjudication of events and monitoring compliance via serial INRs. The mechanism underlying these results remains unclear. It should be noted that patients receiving oral vitamin K antagonists had therapeutic INRs only 46% of the time, which is not uncommon in trials using Coumadin in cancer patients due to comorbid conditions and drug interactions. While a component of the reduction in VTE recurrence can be attributed to increased time within the therapeutic window in the LMWH group, other studies have also raised the question of an impact of LMWH on the tumor biology itself [JCO 2004; 22:1944]. While the CLOT trial initially showed no impact on mortality, a post-hoc analysis at 12 months of follow-up showed a statistically significant reduction in mortality in the subset of patients with non-metastatic cancer [JCO 2005;23: 2123]. A meta-analysis of 7 RCTs comparing long-term LMWH and vitamin K antagonists showed an overall reduction in venous thrombolic events, but no impact on mortality. [*Cochrane Database Syst Rev.* 2011; CD006650]

THROMBOPHILIA, CLINICAL FACTORS, AND RECURRENT VENOUS THROMBOTIC EVENTS
Christiansen SC, Cannegieter SC, Koster T, et al.
Journal of the American Medical Association. 2005; 293: 2352

Summary: The greatest predictor of a venous thrombotic event is a prior venous thombosis, not the presence of a prothrombotic laboratory abnormality. Additional risk factors include birth control medication, male sex, ≥2 prothrombotic abnormalities, or an idiopathic first event.

Introduction: After an initial venous thrombotic event (VTE), the rate of recurrence is high (~25% in 5 years) and related to multiple factors, both genetic and environmental. The effect of individual factors on recurrence risk remains unclear.

Objective: "To estimate the recurrence rate of thrombotic events in patients after a first thrombotic event and its determinants, including thrombophilic abnormalities."

Methods
Trial Design: Prospective cohort, The Netherlands
Participants: Consecutive patients with first VTE between 1988-92; Excluded: known malignancy, age >70 or <18
Interventions: Screening for prothrombotic abnormalities (Factor V Leiden, Prothrombin mutation, Factor VIII, IX, XI, fibrinogen, Protein C, S, and AT, homocysteine)
Outcomes: Recurrent VTE (upper or lower extremity venous thrombosis); PE by positive perfusion lung scan, intermediate or high probability V/Q scan, or CT)
Sample size: 474
Randomization: N/A
Blinding: Laboratory technicians were blinded
Statistical methods: Kaplan-Meier, Cox proportional hazards model.

Results
Participant flow: 474 enrolled; 455 completed first questionnaire, 427 the second, 361 the third, 292 completed study. Mean follow-up 7.3yr

Baseline data: 272 women, 202 men
Outcomes and estimation: 2.6% annual risk of recurrence; men > women (HR 2.7 [95% CI 1.8-4.2]). Patients with 0 lab abnormalities had an incidence rate of 22/1000 patient-years; with 1 abnormality 25/1000 pt-yrs (HR 1.2 [0.7-2.1]), with >1 abnormality 30/1000 pt-yrs (HR 1.6 [1.0-2.7]). Hyperfibrinogenemia was the only single lab abnormality to increase risk (HR 1.7 [1.1-2.8]). Patients with an idiopathic first event were more likely to recur (33.2/1000 pt-yrs; vs. provoked 17.7/1000 pt-yrs, HR 1.9 [1.2-2.9]). If idiopathic, there was no difference between having a lab abnormality and not. Women previously on oral contraceptive pills (OCPs) had a higher recurrence rate with resumed OCP use (28 vs 12.9/1000 pt-yrs).
Anticoagulation during followup: 57/474 (12%) received anticoagulant for >12 mos. Of those, 79% had 1 or more prothrombotic abnormalities. Patients with protein C/S/AT deficiencies more likely received prolonged anticoagulation.
Ancillary analyses: No significant difference in ipsilateral vs. contralateral site of recurrent DVT. 319/474 patients (67%) had at least 1 prothrombotic lab abnormality.

Discussion
Conclusion: Male sex, the use of OCPs, and an idiopathic initial thrombotic event all increased the likelihood of VTE recurrence. Clinical factors were more predictive than laboratory findings.
Limitations: A lower risk recurrence was seen in patients with prothrombotic labs than in previous studies, thought related to sample size, follow-up.

Commentary   *Andrew Brunner, MD, Resident in Internal Medicine*
This article provides a large, prospective analysis regarding the risk of recurrent VTE after provoked and unprovoked DVT. Recurrence is highest following unprovoked events, regardless of the presence of an underlying thrombophilic condition. In addition, the presence of a thrombophilic condition does not predict VTE recurrence after stopping anticoagulation [Lancet 2003;362:523]. Notably, patients older than 70 and those with malignancy were excluded and anti-phospholipid antibody syndromes were not evaluated. There was a trend toward an increased rate of recurrence in those with Protein C/S and antithrombin deficiencies (RR 1.8 [CI 0.9-3.7]), who were also more likely to receive prolonged anticoagulation. Thus, it is possible that Protein C/S/AT deficiencies may independently confer an increased risk of recurrence. Although specific thrombophilias are contributors to VTE, this study found their presence to contribute only slightly to the overall VTE recurrence risk while the highest risk was having an initial idiopathic event. Collectively, these findings raise doubts about the clinical benefit of routine testing for an intrinsic prothrombotic state in patients with a VTE.

COMPARISON OF PLASMA EXCHANGE WITH PLASMA INFUSION IN THE TREATMENT OF THROMBOTIC
THROMBOCYTOPENIC PURPURA
Rock GA, Shumak KH, Buskard NA et al.
New England Journal of Medicine. 1991; 325: 393

Summary: Plasmapharesis improves mortality compared to plasma infusion in treating TTP

Introduction: At the time of this study, thrombotic thrombocytopenia purpura (TTP) had a high mortality rate—up to 90%— and the comparative effectiveness of plasma exchange and infusion was unknown.

Objective: "[To compare] plasma exchange with plasma infusion for the treatment of TTP ... The intent was not only to determine which therapy was more effective, but also to obtain a more precise picture of the prognosis for patients with TTP treated with these modern protocols."

Methods
Trial Design: Randomized, multicenter trial in Canada including 16 sites
Participants: Patients with thrombocytopenia [Platelet (Plt) <100K] and evidence of hemolytic anemia on peripheral blood smear. Excluded: known etiology of hemolytic anemia (e.g., disseminated intravascular coagulation), or contraindication to plasma infusion in treating physician's opinion (e.g., CHF, anuria)
Interventions: Exchange: 1.5 times anticipated plasma volume of plasma infusion for initial 3 days, then 1x times thereafter. Infusion: 30 cc/kg on first day, then 15 ml/kg thereafter for 7 days. Intervention was tapered if successful (Plt>150K for two days) following initial cycle. Otherwise, intervention was repeated or if patient deteriorated, crossover from infusion to exchange was permitted. Patients were also treated with ASA 325 mg and dipyridamole 400 mg PO for two weeks.
Outcomes: Assessed after finishing first cycle (day 9) and at 6 months. Included mortality, absolute plate count, increase in platelet count, neurologic status
Sample size: 100; powered to detect 20% difference in treatment response at alpha = 0.05
Blinding: Unblinded

Statistical methods: 95% confidence intervals, the exact binomial test, and survival analysis with the Breslow-Gehan test
Results
Participant flow: 102 patients randomized after one dropout due to rapid improvement in condition
Baseline data: Groups similar
Outcomes and estimation: At 9 days: both treatment success (47% vs. 25%; p=0.025) and mortality (4% vs. 16%; p – 0.025) improved with exchange vs. infusion. At 6 months trends continued, with an ARR in mortality of 15.6% (21.6% vs. 37.2%; p = 0.036). High crossover rate from infusion to exchange group after first treatment cycle.
Ancillary analyses: Both procedures well tolerated; on patient in plasma exchange arm died of GI bleeding

Discussion
Conclusion: Plasma exchange lead to greater treatment success and improved mortality compared with plasma exchange.

Limitations: Criteria for TTP may have been non-specific; excluded patients with renal failure due to concerns of volume overload in infusion arm

Funding: National Health Research and Development Program, Canada

---

Commentary   *Jonathan Soverow, MD, MPH, Resident in Internal Medicine*
This was the first large randomized trial to directly compare plasma exchange with infusion –the two most widely used treatments for TTP at the time— and affirmed the supremacy of plasma exchange, which provided an early and sustained mortality benefit. TTP typically results from a deficiency of or autoimmune interference with the protease ADAMTS13, which cleaves von Willebrand factor multimers. Plasma infusion is most beneficial in patients with congenital TTP, but patients with acquired TTP, as demonstrated in this study, strongly benefit from plasma exchange, which will remove those antibodies affecting ADAMTS13. To prevent further antibody production and in patients with relapsed acquired TTP, immunosuppression with steroids or rituximab has been used with limited success, although a large phase III trial (the STAR study) evaluating these adjunctive therapies was stopped early due to poor enrollment.

INITIAL TREATMENT OF IMMUNE THROMBOCYTOPENIC PURPURA WITH HIGH-DOSE
DEXAMETHASONE
Cheng, Y, Wong, R, Soo,Y. et.al.
New England Journal of Medicine. 2003; 349: 831

Summary: A short course of high-dose oral dexamethasone achieves an initial response in 85% of patients
with newly diagnosed immune thrombocytopenic purpura.

Introduction: Corticosteroids are commonly
employed for the initial treatment of immune
thrombocytopenic purpura (ITP). Long-term
corticosteroid therapy, however, has a low rate of
sustained response, and carries a risk of serious
side-effects. The use of short-term, high-dose
dexamethasone for ITP showed promising
outcomes in some small studies.

Objective: "To assess the effectiveness of high-
dose dexamethasone as initial treatment in a series
of consecutive adults with immune
thrombocytopenic purpura."

Methods
Trial Design: Prospective, single-center (Hong
Kong), cohort study
Participants: Adults with newly diagnosed ITP
with platelets (Plt) <20K or Plt<50K and
significant mucosal bleeding. Excluded: relapsed
ITP, corticosteroid treatment within 6mo, history
of significant adverse event with prior
corticosteroids, uncontrolled HTN or diabetes,
active infection, pregnancy
Interventions: 40 mg oral dexamethasone for 4
consecutive days. If there was no initial response,
patients were offered other treatment. If after an
initial response Plt dropped below 30K within 6
months, repeat four-day course of dexamethasone
was given followed by prednisone taper.
Outcomes: Initial response: increase in Plt count
by ≥30K, Plt >50K by day 10 of the study, and
cessation of bleeding. Unresponsiveness: increase
in Plt <30K or Plt <50K by day 10. Sustained
response: Plt >50K at 6 months.

Statistical methods: Student's t-test or Chi-
squared test.
Blinding: Unblinded

Results
Participant flow: 157 patients were diagnosed
with ITP in study period; 32 were excluded; 125
were enrolled in the trial, none lost to follow-up.
Median follow-up 30.5mo
Outcomes and estimation: 85% of patients
achieved initial response, of whom 50% had a
sustained response. All patients with relapse had
initial response to second round of dexamethasone
plus prednisone taper; but approximately half of
these patients required other therapeutic
approaches to maintain Plt >50K. Overall, 36% of
patients required additional therapies.
Ancillary analyses: Median time to relapse was
45d. There was a significant difference in mean
platelet count at 10 days in patients with sustained
response vs. those with subsequent relapse:
132,600± 41,900 vs. 84,700 ± 37,000 Plt/mm³,
respectively. There was a 70% relapse rate in those
with Plt <90K at 10d vs. <20% in those with
Plt>120K at 10d.
Harms: None reported

Discussion
Conclusion: An initial treatment strategy of 4d of
40mg of oral dexamethasone is effective for ITP in
adults.
Limitations: Unblinded study; single treatment
arm; lack of randomization. Over a third of
patients required additional therapies.

Funding: Not specified

Commentary   *Daria Babushok, MD, PhD, Resident in Internal Medicine*
Prior to this publication, the conventional approach to the treatment of ITP had been to use daily
prednisone at 1-2mg/kg, with treatment lasting weeks. Response rates were modest but associated with
complications from high doses of glucocorticoids (hyperglycemia, infection, etc.). This study provides
evidence that a short course of high-dose glucocorticoids can be an effective initial therapeutic approach in
ITP; however, large, randomized controlled studies of high-dose corticosteroids are still needed. To date,
there has not been a randomized trial directly comparing dexamethasone to prednisone in ITP treatment.
Although glucocorticoids are often initially beneficial, this study also illustrates the fraction of patients who
are either refractory to initial steroid therapy (15% in this series) or do not achieve a sustained, complete
response with steroids (36% in this series). Intravenous immunoglobulin (IVIg) has been investigated as an
alternative with data indicating a similar benefit to steroids [Lancet 2002;359:23], but IVIg use is typically
reserved as a supplement to steroids for refractory thrombocytopenia and bleeding. At present, three
primary alternatives in cases of glucocorticoid failure exist: 1) splenectomy [Blood 2004;104:2623; Blood
2008;112:999], 2) rituximab [Blood 2010;115:2755], or 3) thrombopoiesis-stimulating agents [NEJM 2010;363:1889].

ALL-*TRANS*-RETINOIC ACID IN ACUTE PROMYELOCYTIC LEUKEMIA
Tallman MS, Andersen JW, Schiffer CA, et al.
New England Journal of Medicine. 1997; 337: 1021

Summary: The use of all-*trans*-retinoic acid (ATRA) in patients with acute promyelocytic leukemia increases survival rates compared to standard chemotherapy.

Introduction: Acute promyelocytic leukemia (APML) is a subtype of acute myeloid leukemia (AML) associated with high mortality from disseminated intravascular coagulopathy (DIC). APML results from chromosomal translocation t(15:17), producing a fusion protein that inhibits myeloid precursors maturation. ATRA degrades PML-RARα, allowing differentiation of these blasts. However, the disease invariably relapses without continued therapy. The optimal treatment for APML and the best strategy for using ATRA during treatment are unknown.

Objective: "To [1] compare the rates of complete remission, disease-free survival, overall survival, and toxic effects associated with all-*trans*-retinoic acid therapy with those associated with conventional chemotherapy in patients with previously untreated acute promyelocytic leukemia and [2] to determine the value of maintenance therapy with all-*trans*-retinoic acid."

Methods:
Trial Design: Randomized, multicenter (6 groups in US and Canada)
Participants: APML diagnosed on bone marrow (reviewed centrally), no prior chemo (except hydrea), ECOG PS 0-3, normal hepatic and renal function.
Interventions:

Induction		Consolidation			Maintenance
		Cycle 1	Cycle 2		
7+3*	→	7+3*	HiDAC† + daunorubicin	Randomization	ATRA x 1yr
ATRA x 90 days or until CR	→	ATRA x 90 days	HiDAC† + daunorubicin		Observation

*7+3 = danunorubicin on days 1-3, cytarabine on 1-7;
†HiDAC = high dose intermittent Cytarabine
Sample size: 401
Randomization: Not specified

Statistical methods: Intention-to-treat analysis; Fisher's exact test; Kaplan-Meier curves for disease free survival (DFS) and overall survival (OS) at 1-3 years.

Results
Participant flow: 401 enrolled and randomized; 55 patients excluded from detailed analysis. 15 ATRA patients switched to chemo due to toxicities or resistant disease. 229/244 patients in complete remission (CR) underwent consolidation. 199 patients then were randomized to maintenance therapy with ATRA vs. observation
Baseline data: no significant differences
Outcomes and estimation: 1, 2, and 3 year DFS highest in ATRA followed by ATRA maintenance (86%, 75%, 75%); chemo followed by ATRA (77%, 61%, 55%), ATRA followed by obs (75%, 60%, 60%), chemo followed by obs (29%, 18%, 18%). OS was higher in induction with ATRA (84%, 74%, 71%) compared to chemo (75, 57, 50%)
Ancillary analyses: ATRA and chemo induction produce similar CR rates (72% vs. 69%)
Harms: 45/172 (26%) patients treated with ATRA induction developed ATRA syndrome. Two patients (2% of those who received ATRA) died from complications attributable to ATRA syndrome (dyspnea, fever, pulmonary infiltrates, hypotension).

Discussion
Conclusion: Induction or maintenance therapy with ATRA enhances OS and DFS compared to chemotherapy. It is unclear if maintenance ATRA delays or prevents relapse.
Limitations: Chemo had a lower DFS (18% at 3 years) than expected. There were lower CR rates with ATRA than seen previously (72% vs. 91%), attributed to more stringent CR criteria. They did not combine ATRA with chemotherapy, as done in other studies.

Funding: Public Health Service grants from the NCI

Commentary   *Andrew Brunner, MD, Resident in Internal Medicine*
The promyelocytic variant of acute myelogenous leukemia is extremely aggressive and was historically fatal. However, this paper established ATRA as critical to the treatment of APML and ushered in a new era in the treatment and favorable prognosis of APML. Although APML is rare and comprises only 5-20% of new AML cases, it is critical to recognize the potential for APML in any new leukemic patient and to consider giving ATRA even while awaiting formal diagnosis. This paper also highlights the advent of targeted therapies for cancer – in this case, ATRA targets the pathologic fusion protein PML-RARα – and proves the concept that cancer cells can be reprogrammed to become normal cells. The example of ATRA in APML represents an exciting advance in the treatment and understanding of cancer biology.

EFFICACY AND SAFETY OF A SPECIFIC INHIBITOR OF THE BCR-ABL TYROSINE KINASE IN CHRONIC MYELOID LEUKEMIA
Druker, BJ, Talpaz, M., Resta, D., et al.
New England Journal of Medicine. 2001; 344: 1031

Summary: The specific tyrosine kinase inhibitor STI571 (imatinib) is safe and produces hematologic and cytogenetic responses in chronic myeloid leukemia, including non-responders to interferon alfa.

Introduction: Chronic myeloid leukemia (CML) is a form of chronic leukemia characterized by malignant myeloid cells containing the Philadelphia (Ph) chromosome, a reciprocal 9;22 translocation. This generates a constitutively-active tyrosine kinase, BCR-ABL, that is sufficient to cause CML. Prior to 2001, treatments were limited and included IFN-alpha and allogeneic stem cell transplantation.

Objective: "We conducted a phase 1 dose-escalating trial of STI571, a specific inhibitor of the BCR-ABL tyrosine kinase… [in] patients with CML in the chronic phase in whom treatment with interferon alpha had failed."

Methods
Trial Design: Phase 1, multi-center trial
Participants: Age >18, chronic phase CML, Ph chromosome positive, failed IFN-alpha. Excluded: plt < 10,000/mm³, 'inadequate' renal, hepatic, cardiac function and poor performance status
Interventions: Dose escalation (25-1000 mg/day) of STI571 to each participant; 14 dose cohorts
Outcomes: Safety and tolerability of STI571. Secondary: antileukemic activity, assessed by hematologic response (reduction in WBC) and cytogenetic response (reduction of cells containing Ph chromosome in bone marrow).
Sample size: 83 patients
Randomization: None
Blinding: None
Statistical methods: Concentration time curves were analyzed by a non-compartmental analysis.

Results
Participant flow: 83 patients received STI571 in 1 of 14 dose cohorts; dose escalation among cohorts; 2 patients stopped therapy due to angina (1) and rash (1). Data represent an interim analysis.
Baseline data: Male (66%); median age 55
Outcomes and estimation: STI571 was well tolerated with no maximal tolerated dose found. Common side effects: nausea (43%), myalgias (41%), edema (39%) and diarrhea (25%). Hematologic responses occurred in 93% of all patients and 100% of patients receiving ≥140mg. A cytogenetic response occurred in 54% of patients receiving ≥300mg. Of patients with cytogenetic responses in this dose range, 31% experienced a major response and 13% had a complete response. Response rates occurred in a dose dependent manner.
Ancillary analyses: BCR-ABL kinase inhibition was dose-dependent with a plateau effect at 250-750 mg daily and no effect seen at 25-50 mg daily.
Harms: As above. No reported deaths.

Discussion
Conclusion: STI571, an oral, specific inhibitor of the BCR-ABL tyrosine kinase, was well tolerated and had substantial activity against CML in patients with late stage disease.
Limitations: Open label, non-randomized trial

Funding: Supported by the National Cancer Institute and Novartis Pharmaceuticals (makers of imatinib, also known as Gleevec).

Commentary   *Sheheryar Kabraji, BM BCh, MA, Resident in Internal Medicine*
In this landmark publication, Druker and colleagues demonstrated the safety and initial efficacy of Imatinib as a prelude to its establishment as first line therapy for chronic CML. The dramatic hematologic and cytogenetic responses seen in this phase 1 trial have been borne out by an 8 year overall survival rate in a similar population of 85%. Imatinib not only altered the natural history of chronic CML but established a new paradigm in cancer research. Since 2001, novel tyrosine kinase inhibitors for breast, lung, colorectal cancer and GIST have been developed by identifying oncogenes involved in each tumor type. The experience with imatinib has also provided important lessons for the future use and development of new cancer therapies. The development of imatinib resistance in CML has led to continued development of new inhibitors, such as nilotinib and dasatinib. Both were FDA approved in 2010 for treatment of CML. At present, imatinib remains first-line treatment for chronic phase CML, with allogeneic stem cell transplantion an option for suitable patients whose disease enters an accelerated or blast phase.

ACTIVATING MUTATIONS IN THE EPIDERMAL GROWTH FACTOR RECEPTOR UNDERLYING
RESPONSIVENESS OF NON-SMALL CELL LUNG CANCER TO GEFITINIB
Lynch TJ, Bell DW, Sordella R, et al.
New England Journal of Medicine. 2004; 350: 2129

Summary: A subgroup of patients with non-small cell lung cancer harbor mutations in the epidermal growth factor receptor gene that predict response to the tyrosine kinase inhibitor gefitinib.

Introduction: A majority of patients with non-small cell lung cancer (NSCLC) do not respond to gefitinib, a competitive inhibitor of epidermal growth factor receptor (EGFR). A small subset of patients (~10%), however, show a rapid and dramatic response.

Objective: "We evaluated tumors from patients with these dramatic responses to determine the underlying mechanisms... We searched for mutations in the EGFR gene in primary tumors from patients with NSCLC who had a response to gefitinib and those who did not have a response."

Methods:
Trial Design: Translational study; case control
Participants: 9 tumor samples from NSCLC patients with dramatic responses to gefitinib, 7 samples of patients unresponsive to gefitinib, and 25 specimens of NSCLC patients who were never exposed to gefitinib
Interventions: The entire EGFR coding region of each tumor sample was sequenced using polymerase-chain-reaction (PCR) and analyzed for mutations. The functional consequences of each identified mutation were evaluated in cell culture.
Outcomes: Clinical characteristics of gefitinib responders (age, sex, histology, smoking status, prior chemotherapy) and location of EGFR mutations. Ancillary analysis: tyrosine kinase activity and gefitinib-induced receptor inhibition in cultured cells expressing mutant EGFR proteins following transfection
Sample size: 41 NSCLC tissue samples
Statistical Methods: Two-sided Fisher's exact test

Results
Baseline data: A majority of patients in this study with a response to gefitinib were women, had never smoked and had bronchoalveolar tumors.
Outcomes and estimation: Heterozygous mutations in the tyrosine kinase domain of EGFR were seen in 8 of 9 responders to gefitinib. Mutations were either in-frame deletions or amino acid substitutions. Matched normal tissue from 4 of 9 patients showed wild-type EGFR sequences. 2 of 25 (8%) NSCLC patients who had never received gefitinib exhibited similar mutations.
Ancillary analyses: When expressed in cell culture, the above EGFR mutations resulted in increased activation and a prolonged duration of action upon exposure to EGF compared to wild-type. However, these cells were more sensitive to inhibition by gefitinib compared to wild type.
Harms: None

Discussion
Conclusion: Activating mutations within the tyrosine kinase domain of EGFR appear to correlate with clinical responsiveness to gefitinib in patients with NSCLC.
Limitations: Lack of prospective validation; small sample size

Funding: National Institutes of Health, Doris Duke Foundation

---

Commentary   *Aparna Mani, MD, PhD, Resident in Internal Medicine*
Advanced NSCLC carries a very poor prognosis. Traditional first-line, platinum-based chemotherapy provides marginal response rates, benefiting less than 30% of patients [NEJM 2011; 364:947]. Encouraged by the introduction of imatinib in CML and Herceptin in breast cancer, attempts were made to identify more targeted therapies for lung cancer. Despite observations that EGFR signaling is over-expressed frequently in NSCLC, previous clinical trials using EGFR inhibitors demonstrated benefits in a small subset of patients. In this paper, Lynch et al. provide a mechanistic basis for this benefit and introduce a genotype-directed approach to selecting which patients to treat with gefitinib. The paper also highlights the concept of the "driver" mutation, in which activating mutations in a tyrosine kinase promotes, or drives, cell proliferation. NSCLC specimens are now routinely tested for dozens of "driver" mutations, including EGFR and the anaplastic lymphoma kinase (ALK) [NEJM 2010; 363:1693]. It remains unclear, however, whether selecting initial therapies based on mutational analysis will result in improved overall survival.

EARLY PALLIATIVE CARE FOR PATIENTS WITH METASTATIC NON-SMALL-CELL LUNG CANCER
Temel JS, Greer JA, Muzikansky A, et al.
New England Journal of Medicine. 2010; 363: 733

Summary: The integration of early palliative care along with standard oncological care in patients with metastatic non-small lung cancer leads to improvement in quality of life, mood, and a longer overall survival despite subjects receiving less aggressive care at the end of life.

Introduction: Patients with advanced cancer often receive aggressive care at the end of life and palliative care is introduced late in the treatment course. It is unclear if earlier introduction of palliative care might improve patient outcomes.

Objective: "To examine the effect of early palliative care integrated with standard oncological care on patient-reported outcomes, the use of health services, and the quality of end-of-life care among patients with metastatic non-small-cell lung cancer."

Methods
Trial Design: Randomized, one tertiary center (US)
Participants: Patients with metastatic non-small-cell lung cancer (NSCLC); Excluded: patients already receiving palliative care
Interventions: Standard oncological care (with referral to palliative care at the treating oncologists' discretion) vs. early (within 8 weeks of diagnosis) outpatient palliative care referral along with standard oncological care
Outcomes: Primary: quality of life (QOL; assessed by Functional Assessment of Cancer Therapy-Lung, FACT-L) at 12wks. Secondary: mood (Hospital Anxiety and Depression Scale and Patient Health Questionnaire 9), aggressive end-of-life care (chemotherapy within 14 days before death, no hospice care, admission to hospice 3d or less before death)
Sample size: 151; 80% power to detect change in QOL with a medium effect size of 0.5 standard deviations
Randomization: Random computer-generated numbers

Blinding: Unblinded
Statistical methods: Intention-to-treat analysis; Fisher's exact test/chi-square test, student's t-test for continuous variables, Kaplan-Meier method for survival

Results:
Participant flow: 151 enrolled, all randomized; 27 died by 12 weeks; 107 completed assessments
Baseline data: No significant differences
Outcomes and estimation: In the intervention group there was: higher QOL (FACT-L 98 vs. 91.5, p=0.03); less depressive symptoms (16% vs. 38%, p=0.01); less aggressive care (33% vs. 54%, p=0.05); and improved median survival (11.6mo vs. 8.9mo, p=0.02)
Ancillary analyses: No differences in anxiety between arms; duration of hospice care 11 days in palliative care vs. 4 days control (p=0.09); resuscitation preferences documented in medical record 54% in intervention group vs. 33% in control (p=0.05)
Harms: None

Discussion
Conclusion: In patients with advanced NSCLC, early palliative care augmented quality of life and mood, as well as longer survival (by approximately 2 mos) despite less aggressive care at the end of life.
Limitations: Study performed at a single tertiary care center with an established network of palliative care providers. Results may not be generalizable or replicable to other types of cancer. Study population lacked ethnic/racial diversity.

Commentary   *Areej El-Jawahri, MD, Resident in Internal Medicine*
This is the first randomized study to evaluate the effect of early palliative care in patients with metastatic NSCLC. Not only did early palliative care lead to improvement in quality of life and mood, but it also resulted in 2.7 months increase in overall survival despite subjects in the palliative care arm receiving less aggressive care at the end-of-life. This survival impact is comparable/superior to chemotherapeutic interventions typically used in this population, without any important side effects. Therefore, early palliative care represents an important and effective adjunct to the care of NSCLC patients with significant disease burden. Although the study's strength lies in its rigorous design and statistical power, its findings are limited because the study was performed in one patient population at a single tertiary care center with a prominent palliative care department. It may be difficult to disseminate this model to community or to achieve the same significant results. Cost of care analyses were also not conducted, but will be of interest. It will take further studies to better elucidate the important mediators of these benefits. (e.g. Does improved mood lead to longer survival? Is the benefit simply a result of more frequent human interface, or do palliative care providers offer a unique benefit?)

MUTATIONS AND TREATMENT OUTCOME IN CYTOGENETICALLY NORMAL ACUTE MYELOID LEUKEMIA
Schlenk RF, Dohner K, Krauter J, et al.
New England Journal of Medicine. 2008; 358: 1909

Summary: There are several genetic mutations in cytogenetically normal acute myeloid leukemia cells that correlate with a favorable response to therapy and survival.

Introduction: Patients with acute myeloid leukemia (AML) cells having normal cytogenetics (no visible chromosomal disruption in the leukemia cell clone) have an intermediate prognosis and it is not clear whom amongst this group would benefit from allogeneic stem cell transplant (ASCT) during first remission. Cytogenetic analysis, however, does not account for all genetic heterogeneity. A more detailed understanding of the clinical impact of genetic variety in AML, even if it is cytogenetically normal, would be helpful in stratifying patients.

Objective: "…to assess the frequencies and interactions of mutations…[and] evaluate the association of the mutations with outcomes…in patients with cytogenetically normal AML."

Methods
Trial Design: Prospective study of patients enrolled in 1 of 4 multi-center treatment trials in Europe
Participants: Patients with AML and normal karyotype on chromosome-banding analysis
Interventions: Standardized double-induction therapy with idarubicin, cytarabine and etoposide. Second cycle consolidation therapy included allogenic stem-cell transplant if HLA-matched related donor was available. If no matched donor, high-dose cytarabine or autologous stem-cell transplant was given. Blood or bone marrow specimens from each patient were tested for gene fusions *PML–RARA*, *CBFB–MYH11*, and *RUNX1–RUNX1T* and for mutations in the *FLT3*, *CEBPA*, *MLL*, *NPM1*, and *NRAS* genes.
Outcomes: Primary: relapse-free survival. Secondary: complete remission after induction therapy and overall survival.
Statistical methods: Conditional logistic-regression model for baseline characteristics; Cox model to identify prognostic variables

Results
Participant flow: 1919 total patients, 872 (45%) with cytogenetically normal AML included in study
Baseline data: 693 (79%) of total patients enrolled had at least one marker analyzed; all 6 markers were assessed in only 50% of the sample; those with ≥1 markers available had significantly higher WBC count and higher percentage of blasts
Outcomes and estimation: Two markers associated with favorable outcomes (frequency of mutation): *CEBPA* (12%) and *NPM1* without *FLT3-ITD* (~35%). Hazard ratio for relapse or death during remission (95% CI): *CEBPA* 0.48 (0.30-0.75) and *NPM1* without *FLT3-ITD* 0.44 (0.32-0.61). For reference, matched donor gives HR of 0.60 (0.44-0.82). 4 year survival for mutant CEBPA and NPM1: 62% and 60%, respectively.
Ancillary analyses: Besides genotype, younger age was the only other significant predictor of overall survival. Type of AML did not affect end points. Only patients with no favorable mutations benefited from allogenic transplant.

Discussion
Conclusion: Two genetic mutations are associated with a favorable response to therapy and overall survival in cytogenetically normal AML. Patients with mutations in *CEBPA* and *NPM1* may not benefit from related-donor transplantation as first-line treatment.
Limitations: Only 79% of patients had at least one marker analyzed and 50% had all six.

Commentary   *Paul J. Krezanoski, MD, Resident in Internal Medicine and Pediatrics*
Bone marrow transplant reduces the likelihood of relapse in several hematological cancers, but the benefit is counterbalanced by high mortality rates of 15-25% [Lancet. 2006; 368:1894]. When a suitable donor is available, prognostic information about the likelihood of relapse is critical for deciding if the risks of transplant are worthwhile in AML. Previous studies have demonstrated that ASCT is not appropriate as a blanket recommendation for patients with AML in first remission [Br J Haematology 2004; 128: 59]. Cytogenetic analysis represents one means of stratifying patients who would or would not benefit from transplant as part of initial therapy. This study further refines our ability to prognosticate and make therapeutic recommendations by using genetic variation in cytogenetically normal AML. Specifically, those with favorable genetic alterations [CEBPA and NPM1 without FLT3-ITD] will likely not benefit from ASCT during first remission. In addition to improving the treatment of AML, this study emphasizes the fundamental role of genetic alterations in the development and modulation of all cancers and highlights the clinical importance of these genetic underpinnings for therapy and prognosis.

TEMPORARY REMISSIONS IN ACUTE LEUKEMIA IN CHILDREN PRODUCED BY FOLIC ACID
ANTAGONIST, 4-AMINOPTEROYL-GLUTAMIC ACID (AMINOPTERIN)
Sidney Farber M.D., Louis K. Diamond, M.D., Robert D. Mercer, M.D., et al.
New England Journal of Medicine. 1948; 238: 787

Summary: 4-Aminopteroyl-Glutamic Acid, a folic acid antagonist, may induce temporary remissions in acute childhood leukemia.

Introduction: In the 1940s, acute childhood leukemia was refractory to most treatments and universally fatal. Previous efforts at treatment with folic acid conjugates resulted in accelerated cell growth and marked disease progression.

Objective: "It is the purpose of this paper to record the results of clinical and hematologic studies on 5 children with acute leukemia treated by a synthetic compound, 4-aminopteroylglutamic acid (aminopterin). This substance is an antagonist to folic acid…"

Methods
Trial Design: Case series
Participants: 5 children, ages 2-7 years
Interventions: Treatment with aminopterin or other folate antagonists (pteroylaspartic acid and methylpteroic acid)
Outcomes: Descriptive individual case summaries, including hematologic trends, bone marrow biopsy results, and transfusion requirements
Sample size: 5
Randomization: None
Blinding: None
Statistical methods: N/A

Results
Participant flow: Sixteen patients were initially treated with aminopterin, with 10 children having a favorable response. Of those who responded, 5 patients were chosen for inclusion in the case series. In non-responders, 4 out of 6 children died
Outcomes and estimation: Qualitatively, children receiving aminopterin had reductions in organomegaly, normalization of white blood cell counts, and reductions in circulating blast cells (no participant-wide quantification or comparisons were provided). Examination of the bone marrow showed varied responses, ranging from absence or reductions in blast cells to marrow hypoplasia
Ancillary analyses: N/A
Harms: Two patients experienced stomatitis

Discussion
Conclusion: Aminopterin can induce temporary remissions in acute undifferentiated leukemia in children
Limitations: Reporting bias, since only positive responders were reported

Funding: Grant No. 250 of the National Cancer Institute, United States Public Health Service, and Charles H. Hood Dairy Foundation

---

Commentary   *Tara E. Albano, M.D. Resident in Internal Medicine*
It has been over six decades since Sidney Farber published this brief case series. The prevailing standard of care for acute childhood leukemia at the time of this publication was mainly supportive, since the disease had proven refractory to all prior treatments and outcomes were universally poor [BJH. 2006; 134:20]. This landmark paper demonstrated for the very first time that a remission, albeit temporary, was possible with the use of a medication alone. While his descriptions of cases are predominantly qualitative, the paper should be viewed within its historical context. Farber's work on aminopterin would eventually lay the groundwork for the development of less toxic anti-folates such as methotrexate, opening the door to the modern-era of chemotherapy. At present, 5-year survival rates for childhood acute lymphoblastic leukemia approach 85% [J Natl Cancer Inst. 2008;100(18):1301 and CA Cancer J Clin. 2008; 58:71].

A Trial of Darbepoetin Alfa In Type 2 Diabetes and Chronic Kidney Disease
Pfeffer M, Burdmann E, Chen C, et al. for the TREAT investigators
New England Journal of Medicine. 2009; 361: 2019

Summary: Darbepoetin alfa used for anemia in patients with chronic kidney disease not on dialysis does not decrease mortality, cardiovascular events, nor rates of end stage renal disease; however there was a significant increase in stroke rate.

Introduction: Treating anemia in CKD with erythropoiesis stimulating agents (ESA), such as darbepoetin alfa (DPA) was standard of care despite absence of placebo-controlled trials.

Objective: "to test the hypothesis that, in patients with type 2 diabetes, CKD that does not require dialysis, and concomitant anemia, increasing the hemoglobin levels with the use of [DPA] would lower the rates of death, CVD events, and ESRD."

Methods
Trial Design: Randomized, placebo-controlled, international, multicenter
Participants: Type 2 diabetics, CKD with GFR 20-60ml/min, anemia (Hgb≤11 g/dl), transferrin saturation ≥15%. Excluded: poorly controlled HTN, prior or planned transplantation, on IV antibiotics, cancer, HIV, pregnancy, bleeding, recent seizure, major surgery. ESA use 12w prior to study
Interventions: Treatment – DPA q2 weeks at one of 12 strengths based on Hgb level, goal Hgb 13g/dl. Placebo - DPA only as rescue if the Hgb<9.0g/dl
Outcomes: Time to death or CVD event, and time to death or ESRD
Sample size: 4000, 80% power to detect 20% risk reduction in primary outcome
Randomization: computer-generated, permuted-block design, 1:1 ratio, stratified by study site, proteinuria, and history of CVD
Blinding: double-blind
Statistical methods: intention-to-treat, time to event analysis, Kaplan Meier curves

Results
Participant flow: 4047 enrolled, 4038 evaluated, 2012 DPA, 2026 placebo
Baseline data: similar characteristics and data, except for less patients with CHF in DPA arm (31.5% vz 35.2% p=0.01)
Outcomes and estimation: Death or CVD event occurred in 632 in the DPA v 602 placebo arm (31.4% vs 29.7%; p=0.41). Death or ESRD occurred in 652 in the DPA arm vs 618 placebo arm (32.4% vs 30.5%; p=0.29)
Ancillary analyses: In DPA arm, median Hgb 12.5 vs 10.6 (p<0.001). HR for stroke was 1.92 (p<0.001) with DPA. DPA slightly increased quality of life and increased risk of VTE. 46% of placebo arm needed at least 1 rescue dose of DPA.
Harms: Increased risk of stroke, VTE.

Discussion
Conclusion: In diabetic patients with CKD not on dialysis, darbepoetin to treat Hgb < 11 increases stroke without improving survival, or CVD or renal events.
Limitations: Baseline differences between study groups

Funding: Amgen (makers of DPA) with an academic executive committee

Commentary   *Meghan Sise, MD, Resident in Internal Medicine*
This is a large, inclusive study that is generalizable to the vast number of patients with diabetes and CKD. The study outcomes are important and raise a need to validate the treatment goals for Hgb and critically appraise the risk: benefit balance to guide practice, especially given the noted increased stroke risk with higher Hgb levels and use of DPA. This study was ongoing in 2006 when the results of the Correction of Hemoglobin and Outcomes in Renal Insufficiency (CHOIR) study [NEJM 2006; 355:2085] showed that treatment aimed at achieving a higher Hgb level (13.5 g/dl v. 11.3 g/dl) was associated with increased rates of adverse events. It is unclear whether lower Hgb targets would have changed the outcomes of the study. There may still be a role for ESA in treating severe anemia in CKD, as nearly half of the patients in this trial required rescue DPA when Hgb<9.

REVERSAL OF TYPE 1 HEPATORENAL SYNDROME WITH THE ADMINISTRATION OF MIDODRINE AND
OCTREOTIDE
Angeli P, Volpin R, Gerunda G, et al.
Hepatology. 1999;29:1690

Summary: Administration of midodrine and octreotide causes an improvement in glomerular filtration rate in patients with Type 1 hepatorenal syndrome.

Introduction: Hepatorenal syndrome (HRS) may result from splanchnic vasodilation leading to decreased effective circulating volume. Midodrine, an alpha-adrenergic vasoconstrictor, and octreotide, an inhibitor of endogenous vasodilators, may improve renal perfusion in the setting of HRS.

Objective: "to assess the effects on renal hemodynamics and function of midodrine and octreotide in patients with type 1 HRS"

Methods
Trial Design: Prospective observational study
Participants: Cirrhotic patients with ascites with HRS. Excluded: recent GI bleed, hepatic encephalopathy, nephrotoxins, infection, HCC, heart disease, diabetes
Interventions: On day 6, patients received either dopamine 2-4ug/kg/min or midodrine (7.5-12.5mg PO TID) and octreotide (100-200ug SQ TID) to increase MAP>15mmHg for 20 days. All received Albumin 20-40g/day
Outcomes: renal function, survival
Sample size: 13 patients, no power calculation specified
Randomization: not reported
Blinding: Unblinded
Statistical methods: means ± SEM, ANOVA, log rank test of survival

Results
Participant flow: 13 patients; 5 received midodrine/octreotide (M/O), 8 received dopamine
Baseline data: hemodynamics, LFTs, renal function, hormonal parameters similar
Outcomes and estimation: Renal function: M/O group had significantly lower creatinine (1.8 versus 5.0 mg/dL; p<0.01), higher GFR (46 versus 10 mL/min ; p<0.001), and increased urine volume (1540 versus 680 mL/day; p<0.001) at day 20. Survival: 4/5 treated with M/O survived to hospital discharge or transplantation, whereas only 1/8 treated with dopamine survived to discharge or transplantation.
Ancillary analyses: Urinary renal tubular injury enzymes normalized after treatment with M/O and increased in patients treated with dopamine
Harms: Minimal side effects (tingling, diarrhea)

Discussion
Conclusion: Combined treatment of M/O led to "improvement in renal perfusion after 10 days and near normalization after 20 days" and increased 1-month survival.
Limitations: Not clearly discussed by authors.

Funding: Nothing disclosed

Commentary   *Meghan E. Sise, MD, Medical Resident*
In this landmark study, midodrine and octreotide have a dramatic effect on survival with Type 1 HRS, which was universally fatal without liver transplantation. However, the study is limited by the very small numbers, lack of blinding or randomization, and absence of clear primary outcomes. Patients with GI bleeding and spontaneous bacterial peritonitis, two common precipitants of T1 HRS, were excluded, raising questions about the generalizability of the findings. A retrospective study of the use of midodrine and octreotide for type 1 HRS compared to nonrandomized controls supports the efficacy of octreotide and midodrine in reducing serum creatinine and mortality [Dig Dis Sci 2007; 52:742]. A vasopressin analog—terlipressin—has also been evaluated for the treatment of HRS in randomized trials and appears to show a potential mortality benefit compared with placebo. [Cochrane Database Syst Rev. 2012; 9: CD005162] At the time of this publication, however, terlipressin is not yet available in the United States.

RENAL OUTCOMES WITH TELMISARTAN, RAMIPRIL, OR BOTH, IN PEOPLE AT HIGH VASCULAR RISK
(THE ONTARGET STUDY): A MULTICENTRE, RANDOMISED, DOUBLE-BLIND, CONTROLLED TRIAL
Mann J, Schmieder R, McQueen M, et al.
Lancet. 2008; 372: 547

Summary: While combination ACE inhibitor/ARB therapy decreases proteinuria, it worsens overall renal outcomes in low renal risk groups and provides no clear renal benefit in high renal risk groups.

Introduction: ACE inhibitors and ARBs are known to reduce proteinuria but long term renal outcomes have not been studied in large trials when used in combination.

Objective: To "examine the effects of telmisartan (an ARB), ramipril (an ACE inhibitor), and their combination used at full doses, on renal outcomes in a large population at high cardiovascular risk."

Methods
Trial Design: Randomized, multinational
Participants: Adults age > 55 with atherosclerosis or diabetes with end organ damage. Excluded: major renal artery stenosis, uncorrected Na or volume depletion, Cr > 265 micromol/L (1.3 mg/dL), uncontrolled HTN
Interventions: Telmisartan vs. ramipril vs. both
Outcomes: Primary: dialysis, Cr doubling, or death (composite). Secondary: dialysis or Cr doubling (composite), components of composites, eGFR change, progression of proteinuria
Sample size: 25,620 adults; subset of ONTARGET trial
Randomization: Block, stratified by center via automated telephone
Blinding: 3-4 week patient blinded run-in to uptitrate study drugs, then double-blind
Statistical methods: Intention-to-treat, Cox regression, chi-square test or t-test

Results
Participant flow: 29019 enrolled, 3399 excluded during run-in. Remainder randomized
Baseline data: No significant differences
Outcomes and estimation: Ramipril alone and telmisartan alone were similar in all outcome measures. Primary outcome HR for combination vs. single agent was 1.09 (p=0.037). eGFR declined least with ramipril compared to telmisartan or combination therapy. Proteinuria was less with combination therapy
Ancillary analyses: Primary outcome HR for combination therapy only significant in low renal risk groups (no diabetic nephropathy, DM/HTN, or albuminuria), and nonsignificant with these risk factors
Harms: As above; hypotension

Discussion
Conclusion: Telmisartan monotherapy has similar renal effects to ramipril. Combination therapy reduces proteinuria but worsens rates of dialysis or doubling of serum Cr.
Limitations: Few with advanced diabetic nephropathy; small numbers requiring dialysis or developing Cr doubling therefore leading to wide confidence intervals

Funding: Boehringer-Ingelheim (makers of telmisartan)

Commentary   *Andrew Allegretti, MD, Resident in Internal Medicine*
This study provided a renal sub-group analysis of the ONTARGET trial [NEJM 2008;358:1547], which made the unexpected claim that combination ACE inhibitor/ARB therapy increases renal dysfunction in patients at high risk for cardiovascular disease. Given the widely accepted notion that reducing proteinuria is renoprotective [Curr HTN Rep 2007; 9:430], combination therapy had previously been used broadly in proteinuric patients to prevent disease progression. Instead, this analysis shows that those at low risk for CKD should not be given combination ACE inhibitor/ARB therapy. Study limitations (not specifically powered to detect renal outcomes, inclusion of few patients with advanced nephropathy [4%], not distinguishing acute vs. chronic dialysis use in composite outcomes) may have contributed to the authors' conclusion that combination therapy worsens renal outcomes in this population as a whole. Still, this study supports the use of single agent ACE inhibitor or ARB therapy and more careful use dual therapy. Of note, in 2009, the Lancet retracted the COOPERATE trial [Lancet. 2003 Jan 11;361(9352):117], which previously supported dual therapy, because of scientific misconduct.

ANGIOTENSIN-RECEPTOR BLOCKADE VERSUS CONVERTING-ENZYME INHIBITION IN TYPE 2
DIABETES AND NEPHROPATHY
Barnett AH, Bain SC, Bouter P, et al.
New England Journal of Medicine. 2004; 351: 1952

Summary: In diabetic patients, enalapril and telmisartan provide similar long-term renal protective effects.

Introduction
Hypertension and albuminuria are complications of diabetic nephropathy (DN). DN is the most common reason for renal replacement therapy in the U.S.

Objective: "To demonstrate that the renoprotective effect of telmisartan was similar (not inferior) to that of enalapril."

Methods
Trial Design: Randomized, double-blind, multicenter (N. Europe)
Participants: Adults with type 2 DM, early nephropathy (GFR > 70ml/min /1.73 m^2), BMI > 25, HTN with resting BP < 180/95 after ≥ 3months of ACEI before enrollment; normal renal morphology, urinary albumin 11-999 ug/min; Hgb A1c < 12% and serum Cr < 1.6 mg/dL. Excluded: any condition other than cardiovascular disease that could restrict long-term survival
Interventions: Telmisartan 80mg daily vs Enalapril 20mg daily
Outcomes: Primary: decline in GFR; Secondary: changes in albuminuria, BP, rates of developing ESRD, CV events, mortality
Sample size: 250; powered to detect GFR difference of -10.0ml/1.73 m^2 or more
Randomization: Permuted blocks randomly assigned at a central location
Blinding: Double-blind
Statistical methods: Intention-to-treat; analysis-of-covariance model

Results
Participant flow: 250 randomized (120 telmisartan vs 130 enalapril); 38 and 44 subjects withdrew from telmisartan vs enalapril group respectively.
Baseline data: No significant differences
Outcomes and estimation: The change in GFR was -17.5 with telmisartan vs -15.0 ml/min /1.73 m^2 for treatment difference of -2.6 ml/min /1.73 m^2. (95% CI, -7.6 to 1.6 ml/min /1.73 m^2). Secondary end points were not significantly different after 5 years of follow-up.
Ancillary analyses: Overall change in albumin excretion rate was small and not significantly different between the 2 groups.
Harms: Strokes (6 telmisartan group vs. 6 enalapril group); Cr elevated but < 2.3 mg/dl (2 vs. 2), CHF (9 vs. 7), non-fatal MI (9 vs. 6), death (6 vs. 6)

Discussion
Conclusion: The renoprotective effect of telmisartan is non-inferior to enalapril in patients with nephropathy and type 2 diabetes.

Limitations: 80mg telmisartan is almost 4 times more expensive than 20mg enalapril; optimal renoprotective dosages of the 2 drugs not mentioned.

Funding: Boehringer Ingelheim (makers of telmisartan)

Commentary   *Opeyemi Olabisi, MD, PhD, Resident in Internal Medicine*
This study shows that the renoprotective effect of enalapril and telmisartan are equivalent in diabetic patients with microalbuminuria. The study's main limitations were the high drop out rate (~33%), only 18% of study patients had macroalbuminuria, and a target BP < 160/90, which is higher than current recommendations. The results may not be applicable to patients with more advanced diabetic nephropathy; however, the results are commonly extrapolated to this patient population. As noted elsewhere (see pg 54), the ONTARGET study showed that combination of ACEI and ARB is superior in decreasing proteinuria compared to monotherapy, however, overall it worsens major renal outcomes [NEJM 2008; 358:1547].

A RANDOMIZED , CONTROLLED TRIAL OF EARLY VERSUS LATE INITIATION OF DIALYSIS
Cooper B, Branley P, Bulfone L, et al. for the IDEAL study
New England Journal of Medicine. 2010; 363: 609

Summary: Early initiation of maintenance dialysis in advanced kidney disease, relative to late initiation of dialysis, does not improve mortality or morbidity.

Introduction: In clinical practice, the timing of initiation of maintenance dialysis is variable for patients with stage V CKD (GFR < 15) and it is unknown whether early therapy improves outcomes..

Objective: "To determine whether initiating dialysis early in people with stage V CKD reduces the rate of death from any cause."

Methods
Trial Design: Randomized, multicenter (32 centers in Australia and New Zealand)
Participants: Adults with progressive CKD with GFR of 10-15 ml/min/1.73m². Excluded: Age < 18, GFR < 10, plans to receive kidney from a live donor in < 1yr, recent diagnosis with cancer.
Interventions: Initiation of dialysis when GFR was 10 to 14 (early-start) vs. 5 to 7 ml/min/1.73m² (late-start)
Outcomes: Mortality (primary); clinical outcomes: cardiovascular events, infections, or complication of dialysis (secondary)
Sample size: 828; 80% power to detect 10% change in mortality
Randomization: Randomized centrally by computer, stratified according to center, planned method of dialysis and presence/ absence of DM.
Blinding: Concealed from statistical analysts
Statistical methods: Intention to treat analysis; Student's t-test, Mann-Whitney test for continuous variables; Kaplan-Meier curves; Cox-proportional hazards for time-to-event analysis

Results
Participant flow: 2982 screened, 2154 excluded prior to randomization; remaining 828 were randomized and completed the study
Baseline data: No significant differences
Outcomes and estimation: Similar percentages of patients died in both groups (37.6% of the early-start vs. 36.6% in the late-start group, p= 0.75) during follow-up period of 3.59 years. No difference between the groups in the frequency of adverse events
Ancillary analyses: No difference in quality of life during follow up period
Harms: None identified

Discussion
Conclusion: Initiation of maintenance dialysis for select patients may be deferred until either GFR drops below 7.0ml/min or clinical markers necessitating dialysis are present.
Limitations: 75.9% of late-start group began dialysis at GFR > 7 ml/min.

Funding: National Health and Medical Research council of Australia, the Australian Health Ministers Advisory Council, the Royal Australian College of Physicians/Australian and New Zealand Society of Nephrology, the National Heart Foundation, Baxter Healthcare, Health Funding Authority New Zealand, the international Society for Peritoneal Dialysis, Amgen, Janssen-Cilag

---

Commentary   *Opeyemi Olabisi, MD, PhD , Resident in Internal Medicine*
This is the first large RCT evaluating whether early initiation of dialysis is beneficial. It is notable that 75.9% of patients in the late-start group were initiated on dialysis before reaching the target GFR < 7ml/min due to development of symptoms. Because CKD patients in the US at the time of initiation of dialysis are generally older (mean age > 65 vs 60 in this study) [Renal Data System. USRDS 2009 annual report: atlas of CKD and ESRD in the United States], have more CVD (60 vs 40%) and include significant proportion of blacks of African descent (none reported in this study), the findings of this study may not be generalizable to all patients with stage V CKD in the US. The less controversial conclusion of this study is that delaying initiation of dialysis until emergence of traditional clinical indicators—rather than reliance on GFR alone—does not lead to increased mortality or morbidity in a select group of patients.

INTENSITY OF RENAL SUPPORT IN CRITICALLY ILL PATIENTS WITH ACUTE KIDNEY INJURY
Palevsky P, Zhang J, O'Connor T, et al.
New England Journal of Medicine. 2008; 359: 7

Summary: In ICU patients with acute kidney injury requiring renal replacement therapy, more intensive renal support does not improve survival, organ failure rates, or accelerate renal function recovery.

Introduction: Optimal dosing of renal replacement therapy (RRT) in critically ill patients with acute kidney injury (AKI) is not known.

Objective: "To compare two management strategies for RRT in critically ill patients with [AKI] to determine if increased intensity of therapy is associated with improved outcomes."

Methods
Trial Design: Randomized, multicenter
Participants: Adults age > 18 from 27 VA and university medical centers with ATN or oliguria and either sepsis or ≥ 1 non-renal organ failure. Excluded: baseline Cr > 2 (men) or > 1.5 (women), prior renal transplant, pregnant, weight > 128.5 kg, terminal chronic disease (<28 day expected survival)
Interventions: RRT dictated by clinical practice: "intensive therapy" (intermittent HD/sustained low-efficiency HD 6 days/week or CVVH at 35 mL/kg/hr) vs. "less intensive" (intermittent HD/sustained low efficiency HD 3 days/week or CVVH at 20 mL/kg/hr)
Outcomes: Primary: death from any cause at 60 days. Secondary: in-hospital death, recovery of kidney function (CrCl ≥ 20, no need for dialysis) at 60 days, duration of RRT, ICU/hospital length of stay, days free of other organ failure, return to home, no need for dialysis
Sample size: 1164 needed to detect death rate decrease from 55% to 45% with power of 90%.
Randomization: Computer generated, stratified by non-renal organ failure and presence of oliguria

Blinding: Treatment groups unblinded; investigators unaware of aggregate outcomes
Statistical methods: Intention-to-treat, Kaplan-Meier analysis

Results
Participant flow: 4340 screened, 1124 randomized. 29 withdrew (18/11, intensive/less)
Baseline data: No significant differences. Mostly white men in both groups. Baseline Cr 1.1.
Outcomes and estimation: No difference in death from any cause (p=0.47), in-hospital death (p=0.27), or recovery of kidney function (p=0.24)
Ancillary analyses: No difference in return to home. RRT-free days through day 28 and hospital free days through day 60 (p=0.07 and p=0.053 respectively) favoring intense RRT
Harms: More hypotension requiring vasopressors, hypokalemia, hypophosphatemia with intense RRT

Discussion
Conclusion: There is no added benefit from intensive RRT in critically ill patients with AKI when compared to conventional RRT.
Limitations: Timing of initiation of RRT not standardized by study protocol. Over-representation of males. Those with advanced CKD were excluded.

Funding: Cooperative Studies Program of Department of Veterans Affairs, National Institute Of Diabetes and Digestive and Kidney Diseases.

Commentary   *Andrew Allegretti, MD, Resident in Internal Medicine*
This landmark study was the first large, multicenter RCT showing no advantage with higher intensity RRT in critically ill patients with AKI. Previous studies were small and had conflicting results, leading to considerable difficulty in dosing dialysis in ICU patients. While the concurrent RENAL trial [NEJM. 2009; 361:1627] studied only CVVH in a similar population, this study allowed patients to transition between modes of RRT based on hemodynamics, reflecting actual clinical practice. Both studies confirmed a lack of benefit from higher intensity RRT. This study's limitations included: predominantly white (74%) and male (71%) sample, exclusion of those with mid- to end-stage CKD, thus limiting generalizability to a large proportion of patients who require RRT when critically ill. Volume management was not standardized, allowing for variability between physicians and centers. Still, this well-designed trial remains the current definitive word on dosing dialysis in ICU populations.

SALMETEROL AND FLUTICASONE PROPIONATE AND SURVIVAL IN CHRONIC OBSTRUCTIVE PULMONARY DISEASE (TORCH)
Calverley PMA, Anderson JA, Celli B, et al. for TORCH Investigators
New England Journal of Medicine. 2007; 356:775

Summary: In patients with COPD, combination therapy with a long-acting beta agonist and inhaled corticosteroid did not significantly decrease mortality at 3 years compared with placebo, but did significantly reduce exacerbation rates and improve lung function at the cost of an increased risk of pneumonia

Introduction: Though long-acting beta agonists (LABA) and inhaled corticosteroids (ICS) are used to treat COPD, the survival benefit is unknown

Objective: To test the hypothesis "that the combination of the long-acting beta-agonist salmeterol and the inhaled corticosteroid fluticasone propionate would reduce mortality among patients with COPD, as compared with usual care."

Methods
Trial Design: Randomized, multinational
Participants: Adults age 40-80 with at least 10-pack-year history of smoking, FEV₁ <60% predicted, minimal FEV₁ response to bronchodilator, FEV₁/FVC < 0.70. Excluded: current respiratory disease other than COPD, long-term O_2 therapy, long-term (>6w) oral corticosteroids, expected survival <3yr
Interventions: Combination treatment with salmeterol 50 μg (LABA) + fluticasone 500 μg (ICS) vs. salmeterol alone vs. fluticasone alone vs. placebo
Outcomes: Time to death from any cause by 3yr; Secondary: frequency of exacerbations, health status (per questionnaire); lung function assessed by spirometry; adverse events including fractures
Sample size: 3020 for 90% power to detect a 4.3% absolute reduction in mortality
Randomization: Permuted blocks with stratification by country and smoking status
Blinding: Double-blinded
Statistical methods: Intention-to-treat, t-tests, Cox proportional-hazards model, ANCOVA, Kaplan-Meier estimates, log-rank test

Results:
Participant flow: 8554 patients recruited (2370 withdrew during run-in period, 69% did not meet entry criteria); 6184 randomized to 4 groups, 6112 included in the efficacy analysis. Withdrawal rate in the placebo group (44.2%) was significantly higher than that of the 3 other groups. Similar rates of adherence (88-89%) in all groups who completed study
Baseline data: No significant differences
Outcomes: 3yr mortality was 12.6% with combination-therapy group, 13.5% with salmeterol, 15.2% with placebo, and 16.0% with fluticasone; the hazard ratio for death in the combination-therapy group compared to the placebo group was 0.825 (p=0.052). Death rate in combination-therapy group was significantly lower than that in fluticasone group (p=0.007). Thirty-five percent of deaths were due to pulmonary causes.
Ancillary analyses: Combination-therapy group had significantly fewer exacerbations (HR 0.75 compared to placebo), as well as significantly better health status scores and spirometry measurements compared with the other groups.
Harms: Higher probability of pneumonia in combination-therapy group and fluticasone group compared to placebo group (p<0.001). More oropharyngeal side effects with ICS.

Discussion
Conclusion: The trend toward improved survival in the combination therapy group did not reach statistical significance, but combination therapy significantly decreased exacerbations and improved pulmonary function.
Limitations: Higher rate of withdrawal in the placebo group may have obscured effects of the drugs.
Funding: GlaxoSmithKline

Commentary: *Susan K. Mathai, MD, Resident in Internal Medicine*
This study aimed to answer an important outcome question in COPD: does combination therapy with LABA + ICS improve mortality? Though the trend was certainly in that direction and secondary outcomes (exacerbation rate, health status, spirometry, hospitalizations) favored combination therapy, the decrease in mortality did not reach statistical significance. This may have been due to the high withdrawal rate in the study, especially in the placebo group. A Cochrane review supported a mortality benefit of combination therapy over placebo [Cochrane Database Syst Rev 2007:CD003794]. However, ICS appear to increase the risk of pneumonia [Eur Respir J 2009; 43: 641]. A Cochrane review of combination therapy versus LABA alone suggested a benefit of the former in terms of exacerbations but not mortality [Cochrane Database Syst Rev 2007;CD006829]. Thus, the potential benefits of combination therapy (in particular, the ICS component) must be weighed against the potential risks of pneumonia and other adverse effects.

EFFECT OF SYSTEMIC GLUCOCORTICOIDS ON EXACERBATIONS OF CHRONIC OBSTRUCTIVE PULMONARY DISEASE
(SCCOPE TRIAL)
Niewoehner E, Erbland M, Deupree R, et al.
New England Journal of Medicine. 1999; 340: 1941

Summary: Systemic glucocorticoids improve outcomes in acute exacerbations of chronic obstructive pulmonary disease.

Introduction: Although patients hospitalized with acute chronic obstructive pulmonary disease (COPD) flares are routinely treated with systemic glucocorticoids, the clinical efficacy of this strategy has not been explicitly tested.

Objective: "To evaluate the efficacy of systemic glucocorticoids for exacerbations of COPD. The principal objective was to determine rates of treatment failure. A secondary goal was to determine the optimal duration of treatment."

Methods
Trial Design: Randomized, multicenter trial at 25 participating VA medical centers in the US
Participants: Patients age > 50 with significant smoking history and obstructive disease admitted with COPD exacerbation. Excluded: diagnosis of asthma; use of systemic glucocorticoids in past 30d; coexisting medical conditions that made survival for at least 1yr unlikely
Interventions: Placebo vs 2 wk course of glucocorticoids (methylprednisolone x 72h then prednisone taper over 2 wks) vs 8 wk course of glucocortiocids (methylprednisolone x 72h then prednisone taper over 8 wks)
Outcomes: Treatment failure (death from any cause; need for intubation and mechanical ventilation; readmission for COPD; intensification of pharmacologic therapy [open-label systemic glucocorticoids, high-dose inhaled glucocorticoids, theophylline]). Secondary: change in FEV1, length of hospital stay, and death from any cause during 6mos. follow-up
Sample size: Powered to detect 7.5% absolute difference in treatment failure rate
Randomization: Stratified according to hospital with a permuted-block scheme
Blinding: Double-blinded
Statistical methods: Intention-to-treat analysis; analysis of variance of chi-square test

Results
Participant flow: 1840 patients screened with 271 patients randomized in the study; majority were excluded for glucocorticoid use in the past 30 days
Baseline data: No significant differences
Outcomes and estimation: Treatment failure occurred less frequently in glucocorticoid groups than in placebo group at 30d (23% vs 33%; p=0.04) and at 90d (37% vs 48%; p=0.04). There were no significant differences between the 2wk and 8wk glucocorticoid groups.
Ancillary analyses: The most common reason for treatment failure was intensification of therapy, particularly administration of open-label systemic glucocorticoids. Length of hospital stay was longer in the placebo group (9.7 vs 8.5d; p=0.03).
Harms: Hyperglycemia occurred in more patients in the glucocorticoid group than in the placebo group (15% vs 4%, p=0.002).

Discussion
Conclusion: Systemic glucocorticoids reduce the rate of treatment failure in patients hospitalized with COPD exacerbations. There was no difference between two and eight weeks of systemic glucocorticoids.
Limitations: Nonhospitalized patients and patients with recent exposure to systemic glucocorticoids were excluded. Systemic glucocorticoids may have different efficacy in these groups.

Funding: Cooperative Studies Program of the Department of Veterans Affairs Office of Research and Development; Boehringer Ingelheim

Commentary   *Mihir Parikh, MD, Resident in Internal Medicine*
The SCCOPE study remains the most comprehensive trial of systemic glucocorticoid therapy in patients hospitalized with COPD exacerbation. This randomized, placebo-controlled trial showed that treatment failure was less likely in patients given systemic corticosteroids than placebo. The most common reason for treatment failure was intensification of pharmacologic therapy, and the differences between treatment groups appeared to weaken after six months. For these reasons, the authors admit that the primary benefit of early systemic glucocorticoids may lie in alleviating severe dyspnea more quickly and in decreasing hospital length of stay. Smaller studies have supported the benefit of systemic glucocorticoids, but the exact dosing and duration of therapy remain unclear. A later non-inferiority study indicated the equivalence of oral to IV steroids in most patients with COPD exacerbation [Chest 2007; 132: 1741].

EARLY USE OF NON-INVASIVE VENTILATION FOR ACUTE EXACERBATIONS OF CHRONIC OBSTRUCTIVE
PULMONARY DISEASE ON GENERAL RESPIRATORY WARDS: A MULTICENTRE RANDOMISED
CONTROLLED TRIAL
Plant PK, Owen JL, Elliot MW
The Lancet. 2000; 355: 1931

Summary: Non-invasive ventilation decreased intubation rates and in-hospital mortality in mild-moderate acute COPD exacerbation in a non-ICU setting.

Introduction: Prior studies in the ICU setting have shown that non-invasive ventilation (NIV) can prevent intubation and reduce mortality in severe COPD exacerbations.

Objective: "To find whether the introduction of NIV, early after the admission on a general respiratory ward, was effective at reducing the need for intubation and the mortality associated with acute exacerbations of COPD."

Methods
Trial Design: Randomized, multicenter (14 hospitals in UK)
Participants: Patients admitted for acute COPD exacerbation with respiratory rate (RR) >23/min, pH 7.25-7.35, PaCO$_2$>45 mm Hg, after initial treatment in the ED, and within 12h of admission. Excluded: pH <7.25, GCS score<8, pneumothorax, or "inappropriate"
Interventions: Standard care (supplemental oxygen, nebulized bronchodilators, corticosteroids, antibiotics) vs. standard care plus NIV
Outcomes: Primary: need for intubation defined as (within 14d of admission): pH<7.20, pH 7.20-7.25 on two occasions, hypercapnic coma, PaO2<45 mm Hg despite max. FiO2 or cardiorespiratory arrest. Secondary: RR, sequential ABGs, mobility and nutritional status, mask comfort and breathlessness, nursing workload
Sample size: 236; 80% power to detect a 15% difference in need for intubation
Randomization: Blocked per center
Blinding: Unblinded
Statistical methods: Intention-to-treat analysis, t-test, Mann-Whitney test, Fisher's exact test, log-rank test for Kaplan-Meier curves

Results
Participant flow: 236 enrolled, none lost to follow-up. Fourteen-day follow-up.
Baseline data: Small gender disparity between study arms; median pH 7.31
Outcomes and estimation: Need for intubation: 27.1% of standard group vs. 15.3% of NIV group (p<0.02, NNT=8). In-hospital mortality: 20.3% of standard group vs. 10.2% of NIV group (p=0.05, NNT=10). NIV more rapidly corrected acidosis (p=0.02) in first hour and RR over 4 hours (p=0.035); faster improvement in pCO2 (p=0.058). NIV led to more rapid relief in breathlessness (p=0.025), but did not alter length of stay.
Ancillary analyses: Subgroup with pH <7.30 on enrollment had worse outcomes than less acidemic patients in both arms.
Harms: Potential harm if NIV intervention delayed invasive ventilation when indicated. In NIV arm, 26 more minutes/patient nursing workload within the first 8h

Discussion
Conclusion: Early NIV for COPD exacerbations with mild to moderate acidosis led to more rapidly corrected acidosis, tachypnea, and breathlessness and to a significant reduction in mortality and need for intubation.

Limitations: Excluded those with pH<7.25

Funding: Northern and Yorkshire National Health Service

Commentary   *Marjory Bravard, MD, Resident in Internal Medicine*
This study showed that NIV substantially improves outcomes in mild-moderate COPD exacerbation (namely, fewer intubations and improved survival) and can be done outside an ICU setting. Subsequent studies have shown mixed results in identifying the parameters that predict who is most likely to benefit from NIV. Meta-analyses show overall reductions in intubation and in-hospital mortality; those with more severe exacerbations seem to benefit the most [Ann Intern Med 2003;138:861; Cochrane Database Syst Rev 2004:CD004104]. The effect of NIV on long-term clinical outcomes is unclear.

EIGHT-YEAR FOLLOW-UP OF PATIENTS WITH PERMANENT VENA CAVA FILTERS IN THE PREVENTION OF PULMONARY EMBOLISM (PREPIC)

Decousus H, Barral FG, Buchmuller-Cordier A, et al for the PREPIC study group.
Circulation. 2005; 112: 416

Summary: Inferior vena cava filters decrease the risk of pulmonary embolism while elevating the risk of recurrent deep venous thrombosis. They have no mortality benefit over eight years of follow-up.

Introduction: Inferior vena cava (IVC) filters are an important, commonly used therapy in venous thromboembolism, but there is limited data on their long-term safety and efficacy.

Objective: "To assess the very long-term effect of vena cava filters on venous thromboembolism recurrence, the development of postthrombotic syndrome, and mortality."

Methods

Trial Design: Randomized, multicenter (44 centers in France)

Participants: Adults with acute proximal deep vein thrombosis (DVT) +/- concurrent pulmonary embolism (PE) and at high risk for PE. Excluded: prior filter, contraindication to or failure of anticoagulation, indication for thrombolysis, short life expectancy, allergy to iodine, hereditary thrombophilia, severe renal or hepatic failure, pregnancy, or likelihood of noncompliance

Interventions: IVC filter vs no IVC filter; all received standard anticoagulation for at least three months

Outcomes: Symptomatic PE. Secondary: symptomatic recurrent DVT, total clinical venous thromboembolism, postthrombotic syndrome, major bleedings, death due to any cause

Sample size: 800; powered to detect a reduction in the incidence of PE from 5% to 1%

Randomization: Stratified by center by means of central computer telephone system

Blinding: Open study with events validated by persons blinded to treatment assignment

Statistical methods: Intention-to-treat; Kaplan-Meier method for cumulative rate of events

Results

Participant flow: 735 patients screened; 360 excluded; 93 refused to participate

Baseline data: No significant differences

Outcomes and estimation: Symptomatic PE occurred less frequently in filter group than control group (6.2% vs 15.1%; p=0.008), whereas symptomatic DVT occurred more frequently in filter group than control group (35.7% vs 27.5%, p=0.042). There were no differences in postthrombotic syndrome and death.

Ancillary analyses: Known cancer at inclusion was associated with a significantly increased incidence of recurrent DVT. Most common etiologies of death were cancer, death likely or confirmed from cardiovascular causes, and bleeding.

Harms: There were no differences in major bleeding. In the filter group, 26 of the 57 patients with recurrent DVT experienced filter thrombosis.

Discussion

Conclusion: After 8 years of follow-up, IVC filters reduce risk of PE and increase rate of DVT, but have no impact on total mortality.

Limitations: Diagnosis of PE may have been underestimated in patients with filter because of lower suspicion. Duration of anticoagulation was not randomized.

Funding: Ministere Francais de la Sante; Foundation de l'Avenir

---

Commentary   *Mihir Parikh, MD, Resident in Internal Medicine*

The PREPIC study remains one of the largest trials to date examining the effectiveness of IVC filters in patients with symptomatic DVT. The study has a number of strengths, including large sample size, extended follow-up over eight years, and blinded validation of outcomes, and its results have been used to support the use of IVC filters to reduce the risk of subsequent PE. However, mortality was not affected by IVC filter placement, and symptomatic DVT risk actually increased. These results are similar to the initial analysis of the PREPIC cohort after 12 days of follow-up [NEJM 1998; 338: 409]. There are currently no reliable data to compare the safety and efficacy of specific types of IVC filters.

HEPARIN PLUS ALTEPLASE COMPARED WITH HEPARIN ALONE IN PATIENTS WITH SUBMASSIVE PULMONARY EMBOLISM

Konstantinides S, Geibel A, Heusel G, et al.
New England Journal of Medicine. 2002; 347: 1143

Summary: In patients with submassive pulmonary embolism, thrombolysis with alteplase in addition to anticoagulation with unfractionated heparin resulted in less escalation of care and similar rates of major bleeding but no mortality benefit compared to unfractionated heparin alone.

Introduction: Given a lack of clear data, the use of thrombolysis in patients with submassive pulmonary embolism (PE) remains controversial.

Objective: "To compare the effects of treatment with heparin plus alteplase with the effects of heparin plus placebo on the outcome of patients with acute submassive pulmonary embolism."

Methods

Trial Design: Randomized, multi-center (Germany)
Participants: Patients with confirmed acute PE (CT, V/Q scan, pulmonary angiography), with right ventricular dysfunction or pulmonary hypertension by echocardiography, right ventricular strain on EKG or pulmonary hypertension by right heart catheterization. Excluded: age >80; systolic blood pressure <90 mm Hg; recent trauma, surgery, GI bleed, or stroke
Interventions: 100 mg alteplase (10 mg bolus followed by 90 mg over 2h) + infusion of unfractionated heparin vs. placebo + unfractionated heparin
Outcomes: In-hospital death or clinical deterioration requiring an escalation of treatment (shock requiring pressors, secondary thrombolysis, intubation, CPR, emergency embolectomy). Secondary: recurrent PE, major bleeding, stroke
Sample size: 256; 80% power to detect 33% reduction in primary endpoint, but trial ended at interim analysis
Randomization: Block randomization
Blinding: Double-blinded broken with clinical deterioration
Statistical methods: intention-to-treat analysis; Fisher's exact test, Student's t-test; log-rank test and Kaplan-Meier estimates of event-free survival, proportional-hazards model

Results:
Participant flow: 256 patients underwent randomization; 118 randomized to heparin + alteplase; 138 to heparin + placebo
Baseline data: No significant differences
Outcomes: Mortality rates in both groups were low and similar (3.4% vs. 2.2%, p = 0.71), but the rate of escalation of treatment was significantly lower in the alteplase + heparin group (10.2% vs. 24.6%, p=0.004), and this was mostly due to greater need for secondary thrombolysis in placebo group (7.6% vs. 23.2%, p=0.001). Incidence of primary endpoints was higher in the placebo group (24.6% vs. 11.0%, p=0.006).
Ancillary analyses: Event-free survival according to Kaplan-Meier analysis was significantly higher in the alteplase group (p=0.005). Rates of recurrent PE, major bleeding and stroke were low and similar in the two groups. Age > 70 and female sex were also significantly associated with in-hospital death or escalation of treatment.
Harms: One fatal bleed in the placebo group

Discussion

Conclusion: Alteplase given with heparin resulted in lower incidence of escalation of care, particularly secondary thrombolysis.
Limitations: Definition of right heart dysfunction, unblinding for deterioration directly impact endpoint; mortality rates were lower than expected

Funding: Boehringer Ingelheim Pharma (manufacturer of alteplase)

Commentary   *Susan K. Mathai, MD, Resident in Internal Medicine*

No clinical trial has convincingly demonstrated a mortality benefit of thrombolytic therapy for PE. Some reports describe short-term physiologic benefits. In practice, thrombolysis has generally been considered for massive PE (hemodynamic compromise). The question of thrombolysis for submassive PE (right ventricular dysfunction but normal blood pressure) remains controversial. This study of a selected group of patients with submassive PE found no difference in mortality with alteplase therapy, but did find a reduced need for composite endpoint of "escalation of care," largely due to reduced incidence of secondary thrombolysis. A meta-analysis showed no improvement in survival with thrombolytics compared to heparin for acute PE [Cochrane Database. 2009; CD004437]. Another meta-analysis found a higher risk of major bleeding with thrombolytics in unselected patients with acute PE [JACC 2002; 40: 1660]. Thrombolysis may worsen outcomes when given to low-risk patients [Arch Int Med 2008; 168: 2183].

VENTILATION WITH LOWER TIDAL VOLUMES AS COMPARED WITH TRADITIONAL TIDAL VOLUMES FOR
ACUTE LUNG INJURY AND THE ACUTE RESPIRATORY DISTRESS SYNDROME
The Acute Respiratory Distress Syndrome Network (ARDSNet)
New England Journal of Medicine. 2000; 342:1301

Summary: Low tidal volume ventilation in patients with acute respiratory distress syndrome improves survival and increases both ventilator free days and days without other organ failure.

Introduction: It has been hypothesized that patients with acute respiratory distress syndrome (ARDS) may be vulnerable to worsened lung injury caused by mechanical ventilation with high tidal volumes (TV).

Objective: "To determine whether the use of a lower tidal volume with mechanical ventilation would improve important clinical outcomes in patients with acute lung injury and the acute respiratory distress syndrome."

Methods
Trial Design: Randomized, multi-center (10 universities of ARDSNet); conducted simultaneously in factorial design with lisofylline and ketoconazole studies
Participants: Ventilated, PaO2/FiO2<300, bilateral pulmonary infiltrates, no evidence of left atrial hypertension. Excluded: >36hrs ARDS, <18yo, pregnant, increased ICP, neuromuscular disease, sickle cell disease, severe COPD, severe burns, bone/lung transplant, ESLD
Interventions: Traditional: 12cc/kg predicted body weight (from height and sex), goal peak plateau <50cmH2O; Low TV: 6cc/kg, goal peak plateau <30cmH2O
Outcomes: In-hospital mortality, ventilator-free days. Secondary: days without organ failure or barotrauma
Sample size: 861; power calculation not described
Randomization: Centralized, interactive voice system
Blinding: Unblinded
Statistical methods: Wilcoxon's test for skewed distributions

Results
Participant flow: Traditional TV 429, Low TV 432; no dropout or cross-over
Baseline data: Average age 51, most ARDS secondary to pneumonia or sepsis
Outcomes and estimation: Low TV vs traditional TV: death 31% vs 39.8% (p=0.007); spontaneous respiration at 28d 65.7% vs 55% (p<0.001); ventilator free days 12 vs 10; barotraumas, 10% vs. 11% (p=0.43); days without other organ failure 15 vs. 12 (p=0.006)
Ancillary analyses: Greater decrease in interleukin-6 in low TV; no relationship of injury to compliance
Harms: None mentioned

Discussion
Conclusion: Low TV ventilation in patients with ARDS results in decreased mortality, more ventilator free days, and more days without other organ failure
Limitations: Not explicitly discussed by authors

Funding: National Heart, Lung, and Blood Institute

Commentary   *Ian Barbash, MD, Resident in Internal Medicine*
It has long been theorized that injuring susceptible alveoli by subjecting them to high volumes and pressures can worsen the cytokine cascade present in ARDS. This study provides evidence that ventilation according to a lower tidal volume protocol reduces morality in ARDS, and in the 10 years since publication it has defined the standard of care and cemented the importance of avoiding ventilator-induced lung injury in these patients. It does leave us with the question of what is the "best" tidal volume; the study demonstrates that 6-8 cc/kg of ideal body weight is better than 10-12cc/kg, but does not answer exactly how high or low one should go. Other questions regarding optimal means of mechanical ventilation, such as positive end-expiratory pressure (PEEP) settings, remain open at the present time.

COMPARISON OF TWO FLUID-MANAGEMENT STRATEGIES IN ACUTE LUNG INJURY (FACTT TRIAL)

Weidman et. al. for The National Heart, Lung, and Blood Institute ARDS Clinical Trials Network
New England Journal of Medicine. 2006; 354:2564

Summary: Conservative fluid management strategy improved lung function and decreased the need for mechanical ventilation but did not change mortality in patients with acute lung injury.

Introduction: Optimal fluid management in acute lung injury (ALI) is unknown; fluid restriction or diuresis may improve lung function but may also worsen extrapulmonary organ failure.

Objective: "To investigate the risks and benefits of a fluid-management protocol with a lower (conservative use of fluids) or higher (liberal use of fluids) intravascular pressure…in patients with acute lung injury."

Methods
Trial Design: Randomized, 2x2 factorial design, 20 North American centers
Participants: Intubated patients receiving positive pressure ventilation with PaO2/FiO2 ≤300, radiographic evidence of pulmonary edema without increased left atrial pressure. Excluded: PA catheter after onset of ALI; lung injury >48h; impaired weaning or compliance; condition with 6mos. mortality rate >50%
Interventions: Assigned to PA catheter or a central venous catheter. Patients with effective circulation were assigned to receive furosemide or fluids to either CVP <4 mm Hg or PAOP <8 mm Hg in the conservative-strategy group, or CVP of 10-14 mm Hg or PAOP 10-18 mm Hg in the liberal-strategy group for 7d.
Outcomes: Death at 60d. Secondary: number of ventilator-free days and organ-failure-free days and measures of lung physiology
Sample size: 1000; 90% power to detect a reduction in death from 31% to 21%
Randomization: Automated, permuted blocks of 8
Blinding: Unblinded
Statistical methods: Intention to treat analysis; Kaplan-Meier and z test for mortality; analysis of variance, Mantel-Haenszel test

Results
Participant flow: 11,512 screened and 10,511 excluded; 1001 underwent randomization (503 to conservative-strategy group and 498 to liberal group); 1 was lost to follow-up in liberal-strategy group.
Baseline data: No major differences between groups. Average age 50
Outcomes and estimation: 60d death rate was 25.5±1.9% in the conservative-strategy group and 28.4±2.0% in the liberal-strategy group (p=0.30). 7d cumulative fluid balance was -136 ml in the conservative-strategy group, and +6992 ml in the liberal-strategy group.
Ancillary analyses: Conservative-strategy group had more ventilator-free days (14.6±0.5 vs. 12.1±0.5, p<0.001), days free of CNS failure, and ICU-free days (13.4±0.4 vs. 11.2±0.4, p<0.001) during first 28d. Conservative-strategy group had better lung injury scores and oxygenation indexes. No significant differences in the number of failure-free days for other organs over the first 28d
Harms: Metabolic alkalosis and electrolyte imbalances occurred more in conservative-strategy group. Slightly higher Cr values in conservative group (P=0.06)

Discussion
Conclusion: Compared with a liberal fluid strategy, restrictive fluid management to a goal CVP <4mmHg improved pulmonary function and decreased the need for mechanical ventilation without worsening extrapulmonary organ failure in patieths with ALI.
Limitations: Of screened patients, 91% were excluded. Study underpowered to detect anything but a substantial improvement in primary outcome

Funding: National Heart, Lung, and Blood Institute

Commentary   *Jessica Volk, MD, Resident in Internal Medicine*
Prior to the FACTT trial, optimal fluid management in patients with ALI was unknown, and practice varied widely as practitioners sought to balance reducing lung edema with maximizing extrapulmonary organ perfusion. FACTT was the first large-scale study addressing fluid management in patients with ALI. Although the study was negative in terms of failing to show a mortality benefit, and only showed small decreases in the duration of mechanical ventilation and ICU days, it did demonstrate that a conservative fluid strategy is safe in these patients, as hemodynamic consequences were not of clinical significance. Based on this trial, patients who are normotensive and nonoliguric can be safely treated with a conservative fluid management strategy in hopes of decreasing lung edema. It is important to recognize, however, that these targets may be difficult to apply to many patients with ALI as those included in this study were hemodynamically optimized, relatively young, and had few comorbidities.

NEUROMUSCULAR BLOCKERS IN EARLY ACUTE RESPIRATORY DISTRESS SYNDROME
Papazian L, Forel J-M, Gacouin A, et al.
New England Journal of Medicine. 2010; 363: 1107

Summary: Forty-eight hours of neuromuscular blockade with cisatracurium improved 90-day survival in patients with early severe acute respiratory distress syndrome.

Introduction: A previous small study suggested that 48 hours of neuromuscular blockade during mechanical ventilation in patients with acute respiratory distress syndrome (ARDS) may improve mortality.

Objective: "To determine whether a short period of treatment with the neuromuscular blocking agent cisatracurium besylate early in the course of severe ARDS would improve clinical outcomes."

Methods
Trial Design: Randomized, multicenter (20 ICUs in France)
Participants: Adults with acute hypoxemic respiratory failure under mechanical ventilation for less than 48 hours. Excluded: age <18, pregnancy, enrollment in another trial, increased ICP, home O2 or ventilator requirement, obesity, liver disease, bone marrow transplant, chemo-induced neutropenia, pneumothorax, expected ventilation time <48 hrs, withholding life-sustaining therapy, left atrial hypertension
Interventions: IV cisatracurium vs. placebo infusion for 48 hours
Outcomes: Primary: 90d mortality. Secondary: 28d mortality, days outside ICU, days without organ failure, barotraumas, ICU-acquired paresis, muscle weakness, ventilator-free days
Sample size: 340; 80% power to detect a 15% decrease in 90d mortality
Randomization: Concealed from investigators, computer-generated randomization in blocks of 4 at each study center
Blinding: Double-blinded
Statistical methods: student's t-test, Wilcoxon, chi-square, Fisher's exact test. Two-sided P values, no adjustment for multiple comparisons

Results
Participant flow: 1326 enrolled, 986 were excluded prior to randomization; remaining 340 were randomized (178 to cisatracurium, 162 to placebo), 339 completed the protocol.
Baseline data: Lower PaO2:FiO2 in cisatrcurium group (106 vs. 115)
Outcomes and estimation: Hazard ratio [adjusted for baseline differences in PaO2:FiO2, Simplified Acute Physiology Score (SAPS II)* and plateau pressure] for 90d mortality in the cisatracurium v. placebo group was 0.68 (95% CI 0.48-0.98, p=0.04). No difference in unadjusted 90d mortality (31.6% in cisatracurium group v. 40.7% in placebo group, p=0.08). In the cisatracurium group, there was decreased 28-day mortality, more ventilator-free days, more days without organ failure, more days outside the ICU and decreased incidence of barotrauma or pneumothorax. There was no difference in muscle strength or ICU-acquired paresis between the two groups.
Ancillary analyses: No effect of cisatracurium on 90d mortality in subgroup of patients given corticosteroids
Harms: One patient in cisatracurium group developed bradycardia.

Discussion
Conclusion: A short course of neuromuscular blockade with cisatracurium in early severe ARDS decreased the adjusted 90d mortality rate without causing muscle weakness or paresis.
Limitations: Lower mortality rate than expected, making the study underpowered to detect a mortality difference.

Funding: Assistance Publique-Hopitaux de Marseille, Ministere de la Sante, GlaxoSmithKline France (manufacturer of study drugs)

Commentary   *Katie Famous, MD, PhD, Resident in Internal Medicine*
It has been observed that neuromuscular blockade improves oxygenation in patients with ARDS. This study attempted to discover whether this translates to improvements in other outcomes as well in patients with ARDS and severe refractory hypoxemia. The study demonstrated an improvement in the primary outcome of 90-day mortality, but only after adjusting for differences in severity of illness. In addition, the exact mechanism of benefit is not understood, although it may be related to improved ability to deliver lung-protective ventilation or to some other (perhaps anti-inflammatory) effect of the drug. Given the limitations, it is unclear whether this study can be generalized to all ARDS patients. Further studies will be necessary to confirm these intriguing results before neuromuscular blockade is considered standard therapy in early severe ARDS but, notably, there appeared to be little risk to this therapy.

EARLY GOAL-DIRECTED THERAPY IN THE TREATMENT OF SEVERE SEPSIS AND SEPTIC SHOCK
Rivers E, Nguyen B, Havstad S et al.
New England Journal of Medicine. 2001; 345:1368

Summary: Early goal-directed therapy reduced in-hospital and 60-day mortality in patients with septic shock.

Introduction: Using resuscitation goals to optimize tissue oxygenation failed to reduce mortality in numerous trials, but most of these studied patients well after the onset of sepsis.

Objective: To determine "whether goal-directed therapy before admission to the intensive care unit effectively reduces the incidence of multiorgan dysfunction, mortality, and the use of health care resources among patients with severe sepsis or septic shock."

Methods
Trial Design: Randomized, single center
Participants: 2 of 4 SIRS criteria and either 1) SBP <90 after a fluid challenge or 2) lactate >4mmol/L. Excluded: age <18, pregnancy, acute stroke, ACS, acute pulmonary edema, status asthmaticus, arrhythmia, contraindication for central venous line, active GI bleed, seizure, drug overdose, burns, trauma, need for immediate surgery, ongoing chemo, immunosuppression, DNR order
Interventions: Standard hemodynamic resuscitation vs. early goal-directed therapy (EGDT). EGDT included: placement of a central venous line to measure central venous oxygen saturation (ScvO2) with addition of blood transfusions and/or inotropic support as necessary to maintain ScvO2> 70%.
Outcomes: Primary: in-hospital mortality; Secondary: resuscitation end points, organ-dysfunction, coagulation, required treatments
Sample size: 263; 80% power to detect 15% decrease in inpatient mortality
Randomization: Random computer generation
Blinding: Partially blinded (clinicians not blinded to protocol)
Statistical methods: Intention-to-treat analysis; Student's t-test, chi-squared test, Wilcoxon's rank-sum test, Kaplan-Meier

Results
Participant flow: 288 evaluated, 25 excluded or did not consent. 263 randomized. 27 of these did not complete the protocol due to discontinuation of aggressive therapy, urgent surgery/procedure or patient refusal (14 standard therapy, 13 EGDT)
Baseline data: No significant differences
Outcomes and estimation: In-hospital mortality with EGDT 30.5% vs. 46.5% with standard therapy (p= 0.009). Less organ dysfunction at 72hrs in EGDT group (p<0.001). Combined hemodynamic goals (central venous pressure, mean arterial pressure, urine output) at 72hrs achieved in 99.2% of EGDT group vs. 86.1% in standard therapy group (p<0.001)
Ancillary analyses: 60d mortality with EGDT 44.3% vs. 56.9% with standard therapy (p=0.03)
Harms: None identified

Discussion
Conclusion: Implementation of early goal-directed therapy in the first six hours of presentation decreases mortality, potentially by optimizing tissue oxygenation.
Limitations: Single center, partially blinded, complex multi-faceted intervention, potential for more physician/nursing attention to patients in treatment group

Funding: Henry Ford Health Systems Fund for Research, Weatherby Healthcare Resuscitation Fellowship, Edwards Lifesciences and Nova Biomedical

---

Commentary   *Katie Famous, MD, PhD, Resident in Internal Medicine*
Although tissue oxygen delivery is critically important in the management of sepsis and septic shock, numerous studies over the years have failed to show that targeting specific resuscitation goals is beneficial to patients. Some have theorized that early resuscitation is crucial in reversing organ dysfunction before it becomes irreversible. Therefore, this study employed a resuscitation protocol designed to maximize tissue oxygen delivery within the first six hours of presentation, while still in the emergency department. Although the study showed impressive benefits in outcomes, it has many limitations, particularly the partial blinding, and must be weighed against potentially conflicting evidence seen in later studies [FACTT, N Engl J Med. 2006; 354:2564; see pg 64]. Large multi-center trials are currently ongoing to validate these findings.

HYDROCORTISONE THERAPY FOR PATIENTS WITH SEPTIC SHOCK
Sprung CL, Annane D, Keh D, et al. for the CORTICUS Study Group
New England Journal of Medicine. 2008; 358: 111

Summary: The use of corticosteroids in patients with septic shock does not decrease mortality or reverse shock compared to placebo.

Introduction: Septic shock may be associated with relative adrenal insufficiency, though the benefit of corticosteroids as an adjunctive therapy remains unclear.

Objective: To evaluate "the efficacy and safety of low-dose hydrocortisone therapy in a broad population of patients with septic shock – in particular, patients who had had a response to a corticotropin test, in whom a benefit was unproven."

Methods
Trial Design: Randomized, multicenter (52 ICUs in Europe and Israel)
Participants: Adults admitted to the ICU with clinical evidence of infection, evidence of a systemic response to infection, and onset of shock (SBP<90 despite fluid replacement or a need for vasopressors for ≥1h) within previous 72h. Excluded: Underlying disease with poor prognosis; CPR within 72h of enrollment; immunosuppression; chronic or recent corticosteroid use; patients likely to die within 24h
Interventions: Hydrocortisone (50mg) or placebo IV q6h for 5d, then tapered over 11d
Outcomes: Rate of death at 28d in patients without a response to corticotrophin. Secondary - Rate of death at 28d in patients with a response to corticotropin and in all patients; ICU and hospital death rates; death rate 1y after randomization; reversal of shock; ICU and hospital stay duration
Sample size: 500; powered to detect 10% decrease in mortality (800 patients needed)
Randomization: Concealed from investigators; independent computerized random number generation stratified according to study center in blocks of four

Blinding: Double-blind
Statistical methods: Intention-to-treat analysis (95% follow-up at 1y); Fisher's exact test
Results
Participant flow: 500 enrolled and were randomized, one patient withdrew consent; the rest completed the protocol. 233 patients (46.7%) had no response to corticotropin.
Baseline data: No significant differences
Outcomes and estimation: Hydrocortisone did not improve 28d mortality overall (34.3% vs. 31.5% in placebo, P=0.51), nor among the two pre-defined subgroups (39.2% vs. 36.1%, P=0.69, in patients with no response to corticotropin; 28.8% vs. 28.7% NS in patients with a response to corticotropin)
Ancillary analyses: No difference in proportion of patients in whom shock was reversed; time to reversal was shorter in the hydrocortisone group (3.3 vs. 5.8d, P<0.001); no difference in length of ICU or hospital stay
Harms: Increased incidence of new sepsis/septic shock (RR 1.37, 1.05-1.79); hyperglycemia (RR 1.18, 1.07-1.31); and hypernatremia (RR 1.58, 1.13-2.22) in hydrocortisone group

Discussion
Conclusion: Hydrocortisone did not improve survival in patients with septic shock, regardless of response to corticotropin, but hastened reversal of shock in patients in whom shock was reversed.
Limitations: Under-powered. Twenty-one patients received open-label corticosteroids (4.2%).

Funding: European Commission, the European Society of Intensive Care Medicine, the European Critical Care Research Network, the International Sepsis Forum, and the Gorham Foundation.

Commentary   *Rob McGarrah, MD, Resident in Internal Medicine*
An earlier study [JAMA 2002; 288:862] demonstrated a possible 28d mortality benefit of hydrocortisone + fludrocortisone in patients with septic shock and inadequate adrenal reserve. These results were corroborated in two subsequent meta-analyses [BMJ 2004; 329:480; Ann Intern Med 2004; 141:47] demonstrating improved survival in septic shock with low-dose hydrocortisone treatment, regardless of adrenal function. CORTICUS, the largest trial to date, counters these results and, moreover, shows more adverse events with hydrocortisone therapy. The study was underpowered due to slow enrollment, which may have contributed to the negative result, although if anything there was a trend towards worse outcomes with treatment. A more recent meta-analysis suggested a benefit of steroid use [JAMA 2009; 301:2362] and the benefit of corticosteroids in septic shock remains somewhat controversial, although there is little general enthusiasm for their use given the negative CORTICUS results.

A Comparison of Albumin and Saline for Fluid Resuscitation in the Intensive Care Unit (SAFE)
Finfer S, Bellomo R, Boyce N, et al. for he SAFE Study Investigators
New England Journal of Medicine. 2004; 350: 2247

Summary: In hypovolemic ICU patients, normal saline or albumin infusion led to similar rates of mortality, multi-organ failure, and days in the ICU.

Introduction: Fluid resuscitation is central to the care of many critically ill patients. Albumin is a more effective intravascular volume expander than normal saline (NS), though NS also repletes the extravascular fluid deficit.

Objective: To test "the hypothesis that when 4 percent albumin is compared with 0.9 percent sodium chloride (normal saline) for intravascular-fluid resuscitation in patients in the ICU, there is no difference in the 28-day rate of death from any cause."

Methods
Trial Design: Randomized, multicenter (16 hospitals in Australia and New Zealand)
Participants: Adult surgical and medical ICU patients with clinician-identified (and fulfilling ≥1 objective criterion) intravascular hypovolemia requiring fluids. Excluded: admitted post-cardiac surgery, post-liver transplant or for burns
Interventions: IV 4% albumin vs. IV NS used for all fluid resuscitation in ICU for 28 days, rate and amount dosed by blinded clinicians
Outcomes: Primary: death within 28d. Secondary: survival time, new organ failure, duration of mechanical ventilation, duration of renal-replacement therapy, duration of ICU and hospital stay. Subgroups: trauma, severe sepsis, ARDS
Sample size: 6997; 90% power to detect a 3% difference in absolute mortality
Randomization: Centrally with stratification by study center and presence of trauma diagnosis
Blinding: Double-blinded
Statistical methods: Intention-to-treat analysis; chi-square or Fisher's exact test; unpaired t-test; log-rank test for Kaplan-Meier curves

Results
Participant flow: 6997 enrolled, 67 (26 albumin, 41 NS) withdrew or lost to follow up. Follow-up 28d
Baseline data: Higher mean initial central venous pressure in albumin group (9.0±4.7 vs 8.6±4.6 mm Hg, p=0.03)
Outcomes and estimation: 28d mortality 20.9% in albumin group, 21.1 % in NS group (RR 0.99, 95% CI 0.91-1.09, p=0.87). No significant differences in secondary outcomes.
Ancillary analyses: In subgroups, trauma patients receiving albumin RR of death was 1.36 (0.99-1.86, p=0.06), more pronounced in brain injury. In severe sepsis, RR risk of death in patients receiving albumin was 0.87 (0.74-1.02, p=0.09).
Harms: Albumin group received 71mL/patient more pRBC transfusion over first 2 days

Discussion
Conclusion: 4% albumin and NS provide similar 28d outcomes in a heterogeneous population of hypovolemic ICU patients
Limitations: 8.8% of albumin group and 10.7% of NS group received additional nonstudy resuscitation fluids

Funding: Australian and New Zealand health agencies, and CSL (maker of the NS and albumin used in the study)

Commentary   *Marjory Bravard, MD, Resident in Internal Medicine*
Considerable debate has existed regarding colloid versus crystalloid for fluid resuscitation in critically ill patients. A prior meta-analysis suggested that albumin increased mortality [BMJ 1998;317):235]. The SAFE study is by far the largest randomized study to address this issue, and is considered to be a landmark trial in critical care medicine due in part to its large size and the high rate of compliance with the study protocol. In a heterogeneous group of ICU patients, there was no difference in outcomes between albumin and NS resuscitation and thus albumin resuscitation may not be warranted given the increased cost. However, subgroup analyses suggest that trauma with brain injury (where there may be worse outcomes with albumin resuscitation) and severe sepsis (where there may be a benefit with albumin resuscitation) are two potentially special cases, and the SAFE investigators have performed subsequent analyses of these groups [New Engl J Med 2007;357:874; Intensive Care Med 2011;37:86].

INTENSIVE VERSUS CONVENTIONAL GLUCOSE CONTROL IN CRITICALLY ILL PATIENTS
The NICE-Sugar Study Investigators
New England Journal of Medicine. 2009; 360:1283

Summary: Intensive glucose control in ICU patients increased mortality and episodes of severe hypoglycemia as compared to conventional glucose control.

Introduction: There have been conflicting results regarding the optimal level of glucose control for critically ill hospitalized patients.

Objective: "To test the hypothesis that intensive glucose control reduces mortality at 90 days."

Methods
Trial Design: Randomized, multinational
Participants: Adult medical and surgical patients admitted to ICUs with expected stay of > 3d. Excluded: in ICU for > 24h; expected to be eating the next day
Interventions: Intensive glucose control (target 81-108 mg/dL) vs. conventional control (target < 180 mg/dL) using infusion of IV insulin; management guided by algorithm
Outcomes: Death from any cause within 90d of randomization. Secondary: survival time in first 90d; cause-specific death; durations of mechanical ventilation, renal-replacement therapy, ICU stay and hospital stay
Sample size: 6100; 90% power to detect an absolute difference in mortality of 3.8%
Randomization: Stratified by type of admission (operative vs. nonoperative) and region of site, use of minimization algorithm
Blinding: Unblinded
Statistical methods: Intention-to-treat analysis; chi-square test; logistic regression, Fisher's exact test; unpaired t-tests, Welch's tests, or Wilcoxon rank-sum tests. Kaplan-Meier curves presented.

Results:
Participant flow: 40,171 assessed for eligibility, 31,675 ineligible and 2392 excluded; 6104 randomized; 3010 in the intensive group and 3012 in the conventional group. Study treatment was discontinued prematurely in 10.0% of intensive control group and 7.4% of conventional control group.
Baseline data: No significant differences
Outcomes: Mortality at 90d: 27.5% vs. 24.9% in intensive and conventional control groups, respectively (OR 1.14, p=0.02; number needed to harm =38). Lower median survival time in intensive control group. No significant differences in length of stay, new organ failures or days requiring ventilation or dialysis. Mean time weighted blood glucose level: 115±18 vs. 144±23 mg/dL in intensive and conventional control groups, respectively (p<0.001).
Ancillary analyses: Trend toward lower 90d mortality with intensive control among trauma patients (p=0.07) and among patients receiving corticosteroids at baseline (p=0.06). Excess deaths in intensive control group mostly from cardiovascular causes.
Harms: Severe hypoglycemia (defined as <40 mg/dL) occurred in 6.8% of intensive control group and 0.5% of conventional control group (p< 0.001).

Discussion
Conclusion: Intensive glucose control (target 81-108mg/dL) increased 90d mortality among adults in the ICU compared to a target of 180mg/dL.
Limitations: Subjective inclusion criteria (> 3d expected stay); did not achieve goal blood glucose in intensive control group; unblinded

Funding: Australian National Health and Medical Research Council; Health Research Council of New Zealand; Canadian Institutes for Health Research.

Commentary   *Susan K. Mathai, MD, Resident in Internal Medicine*
A prior study in a single surgical ICU showed significantly lower mortality with intensive glucose control (goal 80-110 mg/dL) compared to conventional glucose control (goal 180-200 mg/dL) [NEJM 2001; 345: 1359]. A follow-up study of 1200 patients in a single medical ICU [NEJM 2006; 354: 449] showed no difference in mortality and a high rate of hypoglycemia with intensive insulin therapy, though some secondary measures (renal impairment, mechanical ventilation, ICU stay) suggested some benefits to stricter glycemic control. Subsequent studies failed to find mortality benefits but did find higher rates of hypoglycemia with intensive control [JAMA 2008;300:933, NEJM 2008;358:125]. NICE-SUGAR is the largest trial done in medical ICU patients to assess whether stricter glycemic control improves patient outcomes; it showed a significantly higher mortality rate and more episodes of severe hypoglycemia in the group with a lower glucose goal (81-108 mg/dL) than in the group with a moderate glucose goal (<180 mg/dL). Other mechanisms for the mortality difference remain unclear.

MONITORING SEDATION STATUS OVER TIME IN ICU PATIENTS: RELIABILITY AND VALIDITY OF THE RICHMOND AGITATION-SEDATION SCALE
Ely EW, Truman B, Shintani A, et al.
Journal of the American Medical Association. 2003; 289: 2983

Summary: The Richmond Agitation-Sedation Scale is a reliable measure with excellent face validitiy for describing sedation level in the ICU.

Introduction: A quantitative and reproducible measurement of agitation and sedation is needed in order to develop target levels for titration of sedation. The Richmond Agitation-Sedation Scale (RASS) is a 10-point scale developed to quantify levels of sedation.

Objective: "To test the reliability and validity of the Richmond Agitation-Sedation Scale (RASS)."

Methods
Trial Design: Prospective cohort study
Participants: ICU patients. All patients in the validity study were intubated. Excluded: history of psychosis or neurologic disease, non-English-speaking/deaf, extubated or died before the nursing screen
Interventions: In the reliability study, patients were evaluated by multiple specialists with daily RASS ratings. Validity was tested via criterion validity, construct validity and face validity.
Outcomes: Inter-rater reliability between RASS, Glasgow Coma Scale (GCS) and Ramsey Scale; correlation with reference standard ratings, assessments of content of consciousness, doses of sedatives and analgesics, and bispectral EEG
Sample size:
Randomization: N/A
Blinding: Unblinded
Statistical methods: For reliability: k indices and 95% confidence intervals. For criterion validity: Wilcoxon rank sum tests, proportional odd models, proportional odds regression analysis, and Spearman correlation coefficient

Results
Participant flow: Reliability testing: 36 / 86 patients admitted to the ICU. Validity testing: 275 / 325 patients receiving mechanical ventilation
Baseline data: No significant differences
Outcomes and estimation: Both the RASS and Ramsey Scale showed excellent interrator reliability across nurses, intensivists and neuropsychiatric experts (kappa 0.91 and 0.94, respectively), superior to GCS (k = 0.64; p < 0.001). RASS criterion validity showed excellent discrimination between levels of consciousness (p<0.001). For construct validity, the RASS correlated with onset of inattention, GCS, and with cumulative sedative medications, successful extubations, and with bispectral EEG. Face validity with 26 critical nurses showed 81% agreement that RASS provided consensus for titration of sedation
Harms: none identified

Discussion
Conclusion: The RASS has high inter-rater reliability and face validity across multiple types of health care professionals.
Limitations: The authors attempted to correlate RASS scores with dose of sedatives; however, this was difficult because of variation in drugs and doses.

Funding: AFAR pharmacology in Aging Grant, Paul Beeson Faculty Scholar Award, K23 NIH, Geriatric Research Education and clinical Center, Aspect medical systems INC

Commentary   *Laura Brenner, MD, Resident in Internal Medicine*
In order to appropriately standardize ICU practices and provide a reliable measure of alertness, agitation, and sedation that can be used between patients and over time in individual patients, a measurement scale is needed that provides consistently meaningful information. The Richmond Agitation-Sedation Scale (RASS) was developed for this purpose and was the first sedation scale validated over multiple days of ICU care against multiple other measures of consciousness. This study demonstrated that this method of evaluation was both reproducible between providers and valid as compared to other measures of sedation. Of note, this study was not used to evaluate its usefulness in making clinical decisions, but suggests that RASS may be used reliably to titrate sedative medications.

DAILY INTERRUPTION OF SEDATIVE INFUSIONS IN CRITICALLY ILL PATIENTS UNDERGOING MECHANICAL
VENTILATION
Kress JP, Pohlman AS, O'Connor MF, Hall, JB.
New England Journal of Medicine. 2000; 342, 1471

Summary: In mechanically ventilated ICU patients, daily awakening trials to assess neurologic status and appropriately titrate sedative medications led to earlier extubation, shorter ICU stay and, fewer neurologic diagnostic tests.

Introduction: Continuous infusions of drugs are often used in mechanically ventilated ICU patients to provide sedation and analgesia. It is unclear how these infusions affect duration of intubation and ICU stay, along with assessment of neurologic status.

Objective: "To determine whether daily interruption of sedative infusions in critically ill patients receiving mechanical ventilation would decrease the duration of mechanical ventilation and the length of stay in the intensive care unit and in the hospital."

Methods

Trial Design: Randomized, single center (Chicago)
Participants: Intubated, mechanically ventilated ICU patients requiring continuous IV sedatives. Excluded: pregnant, transfers from outside institution where sedatives had already been administered, admissions after cardiac arrest
Interventions: Daily interruption (until patient following instructions or uncomfortable) of sedatives (morphine and either propofol or midazolam) starting 48h after enrollment vs. interruption at the discretion of the care team
Outcomes: Primary: duration of mechanical ventilation, length of ICU stay, length of hospital stay in hospital. Secondary: total dosages of sedatives, use of neurologic tests, adverse events
Sample size: Initially 150; power calculations not mentioned
Randomization: Computer-generated; randomized to daily or discretionary interruption; also randomized to propofol or midazolam - 4 subgroups in total (all received morphine)
Blinding: Care team blinded to intervention vs. control group, but unclear whether they could otherwise determine which patients were in intervention group

Statistical methods: Intention-to-treat analysis; Mann-Whitney U test, nominal data by chi-square analysis of Fisher's exact test, Kaplan-Meyer survival analysis, Cox proportional-hazards analysis

Results:
Participant flow: After exclusions (7 in intervention group and 15 in control group, due to removal of endotracheal tube or death within first 48h), 68 patients in intervention group and 60 patients in control group
Baseline data: No significant differences
Outcomes: Intervention group had shorter duration of mechanical ventilation (4.9 vs. 7.3d, p=0.004), decreased ICU stay (6.4 vs. 9.9d, p=0.02), decreased cumulative dose of midazolam (229.8mg vs. 425.5mg p=0.05), fewer diagnostic tests to evaluate for neurologic status (6 CTs vs. 13 CTs + 2 MRIs + 1 LP, p=0.02). No difference in in-hospital mortality rate, adverse events (including reintubation), dosage of propofol administered

Discussion
Conclusion: In mechanically ventilated patients receiving continuous IV infusion of sedative medications, a daily awakening trial can lead to earlier extubation, shorter ICU stay and lower total dosage of midazolam. There was no apparent increase in re-intubation or adverse events due to early extubation, although the study was not powered to detect such differences.
Limitations: Unclear whether blinding of care team was successful; few patients in control group (only 18 of 60) had any awakening trials; trial investigator may have improved the care of patients in the intervention group in other ways by examining them daily; limited power to detect differences in adverse events; single center study

---

Commentary   *Neil Ahluwalia, MD, Resident in Internal Medicine*
Intubated, mechanically ventilated patients are generally given sedation and analgesia. Continuous infusion of sedatives results in a more constant level of sedation and may increase patient comfort as compared to intermittent bolus infusion [Crit Care Med 1998; 26:947]. However, continuous infusion of sedatives may result in "over-sedation," thereby making it difficult to assess a patient's readiness for extubation. This study demonstrates that daily interruption of sedatives results in earlier extubation, less time in the ICU and fewer neurologic diagnostic tests (presumably because patients are less likely to become over-sedated if their neurologic status is assessed daily). A more recent study demonstrated that a daily awakening trial combined with a daily breathing trial led to decreased ventilator time, shorter ICU and hospital stay and lower death rates compared to usual care plus a daily breathing trial [Lancet 2008; 371:126; see pg 72].

EFFICACY AND SAFETY OF A PAIRED SEDATION AND VENTILATOR WEANING PROTOCOL FOR MECHANICALLY
VENTILATED PATIENTS IN INTENSIVE CARE [AWAKENING AND BREATHING CONTROLLED (ABC) TRIAL]: A
RANDOMISED CONTROLLED TRIAL
Girard TD, Kress JP, Fuchs BD et al.
Lancet 2008; 371:126

Summary: A combined daily spontaneous awakening and breathing trial resulted in better outcomes than usual
protocols to remove sedation and mechanical ventilation in ICU patients.

Introduction: Previous studies showed that daily
spontaneous breathing trials (SBTs) and daily
spontaneous awakening trials (SATs) – interruption of
sedatives – can each reduce the duration of mechanical
ventilation. However, due to concerns about patient
safety and agitation, SATs are still not widely used.

Objective: "We assessed the efficacy and safety of a
protocol of daily SATs paired with SBTs versus a
standard SBT protocol in patients receiving patient-
targeted sedation as part of usual care."

Methods
Trial Design: Randomized, multicenter (4 centers in
US)
Participants: Adults who needed mechanical
ventilation ≥12h. Excluded: admission after cardiac
arrest; chronic mechanical ventilation ≥2wk; imminent
death; life support withdrawal; severe neurological
deficits; enrollment in another trial
Interventions: All received center-specific, patient-
targeted sedation. Intervention group (paired SAT and
SBT protocols): daily SAT safety screen→SAT→SBT
safety screen→SBT. Control group (SBT protocol):
SBT safety screen→SBT. During SAT, all sedatives and
analgesics used for sedation were interrupted;
analgesics needed for active pain were continued.
Outcomes: Primary: number of ventilator-free days
during the 28d study period. Secondary: time to
discharge from ICU and hospital; all-cause 28d
mortality; 1yr survival; duration of coma and delirium
Sample size: 334; 80% power to detect a 25% increase
in ventilator-free days
Randomization: Permuted-block, stratified by center
Blinding: Unblinded
Statistical methods: Intention to treat analysis;
chi-square test, Wilcoxon-Mann-Whitney, Kaplan-
Meier

Results
Participant flow: 1658 screened; 336 randomized (168
to each group). Intervention group: 1 early withdrawal,
1 lost to follow-up. Control group: 7 discontinued
protocol, 2 lost to follow-up
Baseline data: Time from admission to enrollment:
median 2.2d. Patients in intervention group received
more propofol prior to enrollment; otherwise, no
major differences between groups
Outcomes and estimation: 90% of intervention
group underwent SAT. More ventilator-free days in
intervention group (14.7±0.9d vs. 11.6±0.9d, p=0.02)
Ancillary analyses: Intervention group had
significantly shorter time to discharge from ICU (9.1d
vs. 12.9d, p=0.01) and hospital (14.9d vs. 19.2d,
p=0.04) and shorter duration of coma (2d vs. 3d,
p=0.002), and were more alert at first successful SBT
(p=0.0001). Trend toward fewer tracheostomies in
intervention group. No difference in 28d mortality, but
improved 1yr survival in intervention group (HR 0.68,
95% CI 0.50-0.92)
Harms: More self-extubations in intervention group
(16 vs. 6, p=0.03), but no difference in reintubations.
1.6% more dysrhythmias during SBT in intervention
group (p=0.02)

Discussion
Conclusion: Compared to usual care, a protocol
consisting of paired daily SATs and SBTs resulted in
more ventilator-free days, less time in the ICU and the
hospital, and improved 1yr survival.
Limitations: Unblinded; analgesics were continued for
pain during 15% of SATs in intervention group;
sedatives were stopped for 31% of patients in control
group before at least one SBT.

Funding: National Institutes of Health

Commentary   *Krishna Reddy, MD, Resident in Internal Medicine*
During mechanical ventilation, sedatives and analgesics are given for multiple reasons, including treatment of patient
distress and facilitation of mechanical ventilation. However, oversedation can be harmful: sedatives accumulate in
the body, and the consequent delay of awakening can result in unnecessary neurologic testing and longer stays in the
ICU and hospital. A prior study showed the benefits of daily interruption of sedatives [NEJM 2000;342:1471]. The ABC
trial demonstrated significant benefits of a protocol pairing daily SATs and SBTs. There were more failed SBTs in
the control group, perhaps because many of these patients (69%) were still on sedatives at the time of SBT. The
amount of personnel time needed for the intervention protocol was not described. Some have concerns about long-
term psychological sequelae of sedative interruption, though the evidence is limited.

WOMEN'S HEALTH INITIATIVE: CALCIUM + VITAMIN D SUPPLEMENTATION & RISK OF FRACTURES
Jackson RD, LaCroix AZ, Gass MG, et al.
New England Journal of Medicine. 2006; 354: 669

Summary: Supplementation with calcium + vitamin D increased hip bone density and the risk of nephrolithiasis without decreasing the number of clinical fractures in healthy postmenopausal women.

Introduction: It is not clear whether calcium + vitamin D supplementation reduces the fracture rates in postmenopausal women.

Objective: "to test the primary hypothesis that postmenopausal women randomly assigned to calcium plus vitamin D supplementation would have a lower risk of hip fracture and, secondarily, of all fracture, than women assigned to placebo."

Methods

Trial Design: Randomized, placebo-controlled
Participants: Women age 50-79 with life expectancy 3+ years. Excluded: hypercalcemia, renal calculi, corticosteroid use, and calcitriol use
Interventions: Elemental calcium carbonate 500 mg BID (Ca) and vitamin D3 200 IU BID vs placebo. Concomitant use of bisphosphonate, calcitonin, HRT, and personal supplement up to 1000 mg/day of calcium and 1000 IU/day of Vit D was also allowed in both groups
Outcomes: Hip fractures, other clinical and radiologic fractures (excluding fractures of ribs, sternum, skull, face, digits, and cervical vertebrae). Secondary: changes in bone mineral density (BMD)
Sample size: 36,282; 85% power to detect 18% relative reduction in hip fracture rates with calcium + Vit D
Randomization: 1:1 randomization
Blinding: Double-blinded
Statistical methods: Intention-to-treat analysis with Cox proportional-hazards models

Results

Participant flow: 36,282 underwent randomization. 4.3% of patients died. 2.7% withdrawn or lost to follow-up
Baseline data: Well balanced between two groups. Mean age 62, mean BMI 29. ~52% were on current hormone therapy in each group. 3-4% of patients with T score <-2.5. 1% on SERM, bisphosphonate, calcitonin
Outcomes and estimation: No difference in rates of hip, spine, or total fractures. Hazard ratio for hip fracture was 0.88 (95% CI 0.72-1.08), 0.90 for vertebral fracture (95% CI 0.74-1.10), and 0.96 for total fractures (95% CI 0.91-1.02). Hip BMD was 1.06% higher in calcium + Vit D group (p<0.01). Average follow-up period of 7 years
Ancillary analyses: Hazard ratio for subgroup of compliant patients (>80% of study medications) was significant at 0.71 (CI 0.52-0.97)
Harms: Increased rates of renal calculi in calcium + Vit D group (Hazard ratio 1.17, 95% CI 1.02-1.34)

Discussion

Conclusion: Calcium + Vit D reduces hip bone loss but does not significantly reduce the rates hip fractures or total fractures.
Limitations: The doses of calcium + Vit D may have been too low to see an effect in a relatively low-risk population with a high rate of crossover. Concurrent HRT use may have masked effect of calcium + Vit D. Underpowered study

Funding: National Center for Research Resources, DHHS, GlaxoSmithKine

---

Commentary   *Cindy Ta, M.D., Resident in Internal Medicine*
This is the largest prospective, randomized, double-blinded trial to date that assessed the combined effects of calcium + vitamin D on fracture rates. The findings can be generalized to community-dwelling, healthy postmenopausal women as the rate of osteoporosis was only 3-4 % in each arm. The trial suggests that supplementation with calcium + vitamin D could increase bone mineral density at the hip and reduce fracture rates in the subgroup of compliant patients, but did not significantly reduce overall fracture rates. The study was underpowered due to lower than expected fracture rates, which may have been due to the healthy population of participants and high rate of HRT use (>50% in each group) [JAMA. 2002; 288:321 demonstrated a decrease in rates of total fractures with HRT use]. Personal supplementation of calcium + vitamin D also made the two groups more similar to each other, and thus made it harder to detect a difference in outcomes. A meta-analysis of 7 randomized trials (68,517 participants, including this trial) demonstrated that calcium plus vitamin D supplementation vs placebo reduced total fractures and hip fracture rates, but vitamin D alone vs placebo (400-800 IU) did not [BMJ 2010;340:b5463].

EFFECT OF ROSIGLITAZONE ON THE RISK OF MYOCARDIAL INFARCTION AND DEATH FROM
CARDIOVASCULAR CAUSES
Nissen SE, Wolski K.
New England Journal of Medicine. 2007; 356: 2457

Summary: Rosiglitazone increases cardiovascular risk, and possibly death, in diabetes patients followed for 24-52 weeks.

Introduction: Rosiglitazone is a widely employed thiazolidinedione diabetes medication approved for its glucose-lowering action; however, its effectiveness in reducing cardiovascular events or cardiovascular-associated outcomes remains unknown.

Objective: To "perform a meta-analysis of trials comparing rosiglitazone with placebo or active comparators to assess the effect of this agent on cardiovascular outcomes."

Methods
Trial Design: Meta-analysis
Participants: Adults with >24 weeks treatment pooled from clinical trials, Glaxo-SmithKline clinical-trial registry, Diabetes Reduction Assessment with Ramipril and Rosiglitazone Medication (DREAM) study, and A Diabetes Outcome Prevention Trial (ADOPT).
Interventions: Rosiglitazone (2-8 mg daily) ± metformin, insulin, or sulfonylurea vs placebo, metformin, insulin, or sulfonylurea.
Outcomes: Myocardial infarction and cardiovascular-associated mortality identified from summary data
Sample size: 27,847
Randomization: N/A
Blinding: Variable
Statistical methods: Fixed effects model validated using Cochran's Q statistic to indicate lack of heterogeneity. Peto method for few events

Results
Participant flow: 15,565 adults assigned to regimens that included rosiglitazone and 12,282 patients in the comparator group.
Baseline data: No significant differences. Mean age 56 years old. Mean A1C 8.2%
Outcomes and estimation: Over a 24-52 week observation period, 86 of rosiglitazone-treated subjects had myocardial infarction vs. 72 comparator subjects. The odds ratio for MI was 1.43 (95% CI, 1.03-1.98; p=0.03). Cardiovascular-associated death trended towards significance with an odds ratio of 1.64 (95% CI, 0.98-2.74; p=0.06) with 39 deaths in the rosiglitazone cohort vs. 22 deaths in the control groups.
Ancillary analyses: The odds ratio of MI and cardiovascular death for rosiglitazone was greater than 1.0 compared to metformin, sulfonylurea, insulin, and placebo.

Discussion
Conclusion: This meta-analysis suggests that rosiglitazone may increase cardiovascular events with a non-significant trend towards increased cardiovascular mortality.
Limitations: Summary data without access to source data, few events, short time frames (24-52 weeks), and no central adjudication processes for events with the exception of the DREAM study (5,269 patients).

Commentary   *James L. Young, MD, PhD, Resident in Internal Medicine*
This meta-analysis sparked a national debate over the safety of rosiglitazone and the thiazolidinedione (TZD) class of glucose-lowering medications, eventually leading to FDA restrictions on the drug and its removal from the market in Europe. Since its publication, meta-analyses incorporating new randomized trial data recapitulated the original findings demonstrating a 30-80% higher risk of acute myocardial infarction in diabetic patients receiving rosiglitazone [Arch Intern Med 2010; 170:1191]. In line with the secondary endpoints of the PROACTIVE study that suggest pioglitazone reduces a composite of myocardial infarction, stroke, and all-cause mortality, initial review of Medicare databases suggested that rosiglitazone confers greater cardiovascular risk than pioglitazone [FDA Briefing Document: July 13-14, 2010]. Nonetheless, these analyses were predominantly limited to short-term events. A large randomized trial, the Rosiglitazone Evaluated for Cardiovascular Outcomes (RECORD) released a final, independently readjudicated analysis in 2013 demonstrating no statistical increase in hospitalization or death from cardiovascular causes, similar to the interim analysis over a follow-up of 3.75 years [NEJM 2007; 357:28], perhaps suggesting different risk profiles over longer time frames. The FDA finally elected to remove restrictions on rosiglitazone in 2013.

THE EFFECT OF INTENSIVE TREATMENT OF DIABETES ON THE DEVELOPMENT AND PROGRESSION OF LONG-TERM COMPLICATIONS IN INSULIN-DEPENDENT DIABETES MELLITUS (DCCT)

The Diabetes Control and Complications Trial (DCCT) Research Group
New England Journal of Medicine. 1993; 329: 977

Summary: Intensive insulin therapy slows the onset and progression of microvascular complications in patients with type 1 diabetes.

Introduction: The microvascular complications of Type 1 diabetes (T1DM), cause significant morbidity and mortality. The ability of intensive blood glucose control to prevent these complications is unclear.

Objective: To "compare intensive with conventional diabetes therapy with regard to their effects on the development and progression of the early vascular and neurologic complications of IDDM."

Methods
Trial Design: Randomized, multicenter (29 centers in US)
Participants: Patients aged 13-39 yrs with T1DM defined by C-peptide deficiency. Primary-prevention group: T1DM 1-5yrs, no retinopathy, urinary albumin excretion <40mg/24hrs. Secondary-intervention group: T1DM 1-15yrs, mild-moderate nonproliferative retinopathy, urinary albumin excretion <200mg/24hrs. Excluded: hypertension, hyperlipidemia, severe diabetic complications
Interventions: Conventional therapy: 1-2 daily insulin injections (with adjustments only to avoid symptoms of hyperglycemia, hypoglycemia, or ketonuria) vs. intensive therapy: >3 insulin injections/day or use of an insulin pump adjusted for goal preprandial blood glucose 70-120 mg/dL, postprandial <180 mg/dL, A1c <6.05%
Outcomes: Retinopathy, nephropathy, neuropathy
Sample size: 1441
Blinding: Unblinded
Statistical methods: Intention-to-treat analysis; Wilcoxon rank-sum test, chi-square test

Results
Participant flow: 1441 enrolled. 726 primary-prevention, 715 secondary-intervention, each group randomized. 11 died. 95 women in conventional group received intensive therapy during pregnancy. Average 6.5yrs follow-up
Baseline data: No significant differences.
Outcomes and estimation: Primary-prevention group: intensive insulin therapy reduced the adjusted mean relative risk of developing retinopathy by 76% (p<0.001, NNT=33), microalbuminuria by 34% (p=0.04, NNT=83) and clinical neuropathy by 69% (p=0.006, NNT=15) compared to conventional therapy. Secondary-intervention group: intensive insulin therapy reduced the adjusted mean relative risk of worsened retinopathy by 54% (p<0.001, NNT=25), microalbuminuria by 43% (p=0.001, NNT=50) and clinical neuropathy by 57% (p<0.001, NNT=11) vs. conventional therapy.
Ancillary analyses: Mean blood glucose was 155+/-30 mg/dL in intensive therapy group vs. 231+/-55 mg/dL in conventional group (p<0.001). No difference in macrovascular events
Harms: No difference in mortality. Hypoglycemia 3 times higher in intensive therapy (p<0.001). Increased weight gain with intensive therapy.

Discussion
Conclusion: Intensive therapy with insulin delays the onset and slows the progression of microvascular complications (including retinopathy, nephropathy, and neuropathy) in T1DM patients.
Limitations: Short period of follow-up to detect macrovascular outcomes, crossover of pregnant patients, unblinded trial
Funding: Academic & corporate sponsors

Commentary　　　　　　　　　　*Kelly Lauter, MD, PhD, Resident in Internal Medicine*
DCCT defined the role of intensive glycemic therapy on the development of long-term microvascular complications of type 1 diabetes. The Epidemiology of Diabetes Interventions and Complications (EDIC) study was designed to follow the DCCT cohort to determine the long-term effects of the original DCCT interventions on microvascular and macrovascular outcomes. The 10-year EDIC follow-up demonstrated that, despite an equalization of Hb A1c between the two groups, the benefit on microvascular outcomes persisted; and it demonstrated a benefit of intensive glycemic control on reduction of macrovascular outcomes [Diabetes Care 1999;22:99]. The United Kingdom Prospective Diabetes Study (UKPDS) showed similar results of improved microvascular outcomes with intensive glycemic therapy in patients with type 2 diabetes [Lancet 1998;352:837 – see pg 76]. Given the 3-fold higher rate of hypoglycemia, the benefits of intensive glycemic control must be weighed against the potential harms of hypoglycemia.

INTENSIVE BLOOD-GLUCOSE CONTROL WITH SULFONYLUREAS OR INSULIN COMPARED WITH
CONVENTIONAL TREATMENT AND RISK OF COMPLICATIONS IN PATIENTS WITH TYPE 2 DIABETES
(UKPDS 33)
UK Prospective Diabetes Study (UKPDS) Group
Lancet. 1998; 352: 837

Summary: Tight glucose control with sulfonylureas and insulin led decreases microvascular (but not macrovascular) complications at the cost of more frequent hypoglycemia, in patients with newly diagnosed Type 2 diabetes mellitus.

Introduction: Improved blood-glucose control slows progression of microvascular complications of both type 1 and type 2 diabetes mellitus (DM) but its effect on macrovascular complications is unknown.

Objective: To "compare the effects of intensive blood-glucose control with either sulfonylureas or insulin and conventional treatment on the risk of microvascular and macrovascular complications in patients with type 2 diabetes."

Methods
Trial Design: Randomized, multicenter (23 hospitals in UK)
Participants: Patients with newly diagnosed type 2 DM, aged 25-65, with fasting glucose of >108 mg/dL. Excluded: patients with significant ketonuria, MI within previous year, Cr >1.98 mg/dl, current angina or heart failure, >1 major vascular event, significant retinopathy, malignant HTN, or other severe illness
Interventions: Intensive treatment group: sulfonylurea or insulin with goal fasting glucose <110 mg/dL vs. conventional treatment group: goal "asymptomatic DM" <270 mg/dL with diet modification alone; if further hyperglycemia occurred in this group, patients were secondarily randomized to sulfonylurea or insulin therapy
Outcomes: (1) any diabetes-related endpoint (sudden death, death from hyperglycemia or hypoglycemia, fatal or nonfatal MI, CHF, CVA, renal failure, amputation, retinopathy or blindness) (2) diabetes-related death, and (3) all-cause mortality
Sample size: 3,867; 81% power to detect 15% risk reduction for composite outcomes
Randomization: Central, computer-generated

Blinding: Unblinded
Statistical methods: Intention-to-treat, log-rank test, Wilcoxon, t-test, and chi-square test; survival-function using Kaplan-Meier method

Results:
Participant flow: 7,616 patients screened, 5,102 recruited; 3-month run-in period with dietary and physician consultation; 3,867 randomized. Mean follow-up was 10 years.
Baseline data: No significant differences. Mean age 53.3 years-old; mean A1C 7.08%.
Outcomes: No difference between intensive (insulin or sulfonylurea) and conventional treatment groups in any of the aggregate endpoints. Diabetes-related mortality and all-cause mortality did not differ between groups.
Ancillary analyses: Median A1C was lower in the intensive vs. conventional group (7% vs. 7.9%, p<0.0001). The intensive treatment group had a 25% RRR in microvascular complications (p<0.01), mostly due to decreased retinopathy. Borderline risk reduction in MI (p=0.052).
Harms: Higher rates of hypoglycemic episodes with intensive therapy, with the highest rates in the insulin subgroup.

Discussion
Conclusion: Improved glycemic control with insulin or sulfonylurea leads to improved microvascular endpoints in newly diagnosed diabetics, but no difference in MI or diabetes-related mortality at 10 years. Neither sulfonylurea nor insulin worsened macrovascular disease.
Limitations: Multiple crossovers

Funding: UK, academic & pharmaceutical

Commentary   *Susan K. Mathai, MD, Resident in Internal Medicine*
The previous large-scale randomized trial, the University Group Diabetes Program [JAMA 1978;240:37], found no evidence that improved glycemic control with any therapy reduced cardiovascular risk. UKPDS showed that intensive glucose reduced micovascular complications, but did not show significant improvements in macrovascular or mortality outcomes. Post-trial monitoring of patients (no longer randomized to the initial groups) showed that, though differences in A1C among initial groups were lost after five years, relative reductions in risk persisted at 10 years for any diabetes-related end point (9%), microvascular disease (24%), MI (15%), and death from any cause (13%, all p<0.05) [NEJM 2008; 359:1577]. Subsequent trials (VADT, ACCORD, ADVANCE), however, have failed to show an improvement in macrovascular outcomes with intensive glycemic control initiated later in the course of diabetes in patients with type 2 DM.

RANDOMIZED STUDY OF BASAL BOLUS INSULIN THERAPY IN THE INPATIENT MANAGEMENT OF
PATIENTS WITH TYPE 2 DIABETES (RABBIT 2)
Guillermo E, Umpierrez, MD, Smiley D, et. al
Diabetes Care. 2007; 30: 2181

Summary: A regimen of glargine (long acting insulin) and glulisine (rapid acting insulin) controls hyperglycemia better than sliding scale regular insulin alone in hospitalized non-ICU patients.

Introduction: Few studies have addressed the optimal management of hyperglycemia in non-ICU inpatients with type 2 diabetes.

Objective: "To compare the efficacy and safety of a basal/bolus insulin regimen to sliding scale regular insulin (SSI) in patients with type 2 diabetes."

Methods
Trial Design: Randomized, open-label, multicenter (Emory University and University of Miami)
Participants: Insulin-naive patients with type 2 diabetes for at least 3 months and admission blood glucose 140-180 mg/dL, admitted to inpatient medial units. Excluded: new-onset diabetes, diabetic ketoacidosis/hyperosmolar hyperglycemic state, prior insulin use, ICU admission, steroid use, liver disease, Cr > 3mg/dL, impaired mental status, pregnancy
Interventions: Glargine daily + glulisine three times daily vs. adjustable regular insulin sliding scale regimen
Outcomes: Primary: mean daily blood glucose. Secondary: hypoglycemia, length of stay, mortality.
Sample size: 130; power calculations not specified
Blinding: Unblinded
Statistical methods: Analysis of Variance (ANOVA)

Participant flow: 130 patients randomized. 65 per group. Unclear how many screened and excluded
Baseline data: No significant differences. Mean admission blood glucose was 227 ± 65 mg/dl and the mean A1C $8.8 \pm 2\%$
Outcomes and estimation: Mean daily glucose was 27 mg/dl lower in the basal-bolus group (p < 0.01). Between days 2-6, a BG target of <140 mg/dl was achieved in 66% of patients in basal-bolus group and in 38% of those in the SSI group. No significant difference in length of stay. Only one patient death, in basal-bolus group (p value not reported)
Adverse Outcomes: 3% hypoglycemia (BG <60 mg/dL) in both groups

Discussion
Conclusion: Treatment with basal-bolus insulin resulted significantly improved glycemic control compared with SSI alone with no major difference in episodes of hypoglycemia or length of stay.
Limitations: Other insulin regimens (such as NPH) were not investigated.

Funding: Sanofi-Aventis [manufacturers of Lantus (glargine)]

Commentary   *Taison Bell, MD, Resident in Internal Medicine*
This was the first randomized trial comparing basal-bolus insulin with sliding scale insulin alone in non-ICU patients. The risk of hypoglycemia often leads to hesitation in starting patients on basal-bolus insulin on admission, and studies of intensive glycemic control in critically ill patients have demonstrated increased rates of hypoglycemia and overall mortality when targeting blood glucose levels of approximately 80-110 [NEJM 2009; 360:1283; NEJM 2008; 358:125]. In this study of non-critically ill patients, targeting a more liberal blood glucose level of <140 mg/dL in the basal plus bolus insulin group resulted in improved glycemic control with lower mean daily blood glucose levels without different rates of rates of hypoglycemia or length of hospital stay compared to insulin sliding scale alone. The study was not powered to detect a mortality effect. The study also had a 14% crossover of the sliding scale only group into the basal plus bolus group for patients with persistently elevated glucoses > 240 mg/dL.

EFFECTS OF INTENSIVE GLUCOSE LOWERING IN TYPE 2 DIABETES (ACCORD)
The ACCORD (Action to Control Cardiovascular Risk in Diabetes) Study Group
New England Journal of Medicine.2008; 358: 2545

Summary: Intensive therapy to target an A1C < 6% does not reduce cardiovascular events but increases mortality and hypoglycemic events in patients with long-standing diabetes at high risk of cardiovascular events.

Introduction: The effect of intensive glycemic control on cardiovascular (CV) events and mortality in patients with type 2 DM is unclear.

Objective: "To determine whether a therpautic strategy targeting normal glycated hemoglobin levels (i.e., below 6.0%) would reduce the rate of cardiovascular events would reduce the rate of CV events, as compared with [...] targeting A1C levels of 7 to 7.9%."

Methods
Trial Design: Randomized, multicenter (77 centers in US and Canada), double 2 x 2 factorial design (also investigating role of blood pressure and lipid reduction)
Participants: Adults with type 2 diabetes who have A1C>7.5% and age 40-79 with CV disease OR age 55-79 with evidence of atherosclerosis, albuminuria, left ventricular hypertrophy or 2 risk factors for CV disease (dyslipidemia, HTN, smoking, obesity). Excluded: frequent or recent hypoglycemic events, unwillingness to perform home glucose monitoring/inject insulin, BMI>45, Cr>1.5, serious illness, age > 79
Interventions: Aggressive lowering of A1C levels to less than 6% vs. 'standard therapy' defined as targeting HbA1c levels to 7.0-7.9. Medications chosen according to clinician preference
Outcomes: Primary: First occurrence of a major CV event (composite of nonfatal MI, nonfatal stroke or CV death). Secondary: death from any cause, microvascular complications, hypoglycemia
Sample size: 10,251; 89% power to detect 15% reduction in primary outcome
Randomization: Central randomization
Blinding: Unblinded
Statistical methods: Intention-to-treat analysis; chi-square test, Cox proportional-hazards

Results
Participant flow: 10,251 randomized (5,128 intensive group – 26 lost to follow-up, 336 discontinued intervention; 5,123 standard group – 24 lost to follow-up, 322 discontinued intervention). Mean follow-up 3.5 yr.
Baseline data: No significant differences. Mean duration of diabetes was 10 yrs.
Outcomes and estimation: Mean A1C 6.4% in in intensive group and 7.5% in standard group. No differences in primary outcome (6.9% intensive therapy vs 7.2% standard therapy, p=0.16). Annual rates of nonfatal MI were lower in the intensive therapy group (3.6% vs 4.6%, p=0.004). However, the rate of death from any cause (5% vs. 4%, p=0.04) and CV causes (2.6% vs. 1.8%, p=0.02) were higher in intensive therapy group, leading to study termination after 3.5 yrs. No difference in rates of stroke (1.3% vs. 1.2%, p=0.74).
Harms: Higher rates of hypoglycemia requiring medical assistance (10.5% vs. 3.5%, p<0.001), fluid retention (70% vs. 67%, p<0.001), and weight gain >10 kg from baseline (27.8% vs. 14.1%, p<0.001) in intensive therapy group.

Discussion
Conclusion: Intensive glycemic control to A1C levels to <6% increased all-cause mortality after an average of 3.5 yrs compared to a goal A1C of 7.0-7.9% in patients with long-standing type 2 diabetes and either pre-existing CV disease or multiple CVD risk factors.
Limitations: The results may not apply to patients with recent-onset type 2 diabetes or those with lower CV risk. Did not address specific strategies of glycated hemoglobin lowering.

Funding: Academic & pharmaceutical

Commentary   *Dina Reiss, MD, Resident in Internal Medicine*
ACCORD suggests a trend towards decreased nonfatal MIs after 3 years of intensive glycemic control, but increased risk of all-cause mortality and cardiovascular mortality in patients with long-standing diabetes with existing cardiovascular disease or multiple cardiovascular risk factors. Other large trials of intensive glycemic control in patients with type 2 diabetes, such as ADVANCE [NEJM 2008;358:3560] and VADT [NEJM 2009;360:129], did not find increased mortality. Patients from the ACCORD trial had a higher rate of preexisting CVD, used more medications and had a longer duration of diabetes prior to enrollment. ACCORD did not have sufficient power to detect a difference in the primary outcome rate at the time of the study termination. The trial did not establish whether a specific medication or combination of medication correlated with increased mortality. Intensive glycemic control may be more beneficial in patients without significant cardiovascular disease or risk factors, or with shorter duration of diabetes, but the potential benefits must be weighed against the increased risks noted here.

ONCE-YEARLY ZOLEDRONIC ACID FOR TREATMENT OF POSTMENOPAUSAL OSTEOPOROSIS
(HORIZON)
Black DM, Delmas PD, Eastell R, et al. for the HORIZON Pivotal Fracture Trial
New England Journal of Medicine. 2007; 356: 1809

Summary: Annual zoledronic acid infusions are effective in reducing vertebral and hip fractures in high-risk postmenopausal women.

Introduction: Many postmenopausal women who are at high risk for osteoporotic fractures and subsequent complications including death cannot tolerate oral bisphosphonate therapy.

Objective: "We assessed the effects of annual infusions of zoledronic acid on fracture risk during a 3-year period."

Methods
Trial Design: Randomized, multicenter (international)
Participants: Post-menopausal women between ages 65-89 with 1) osteoporosis by DEXA or 2) osteopenia by DEXA with vertebral fractures. Patients divided into 2 strata: absence (stratum 1) or presence (stratum 2) of baseline use of non-bisphosphonate osteoporosis medications (e.g. hormone therapy, raloxifene, calcitonin, tibolone, tamoxifen, dehydroepiandrosterone, ipriflavone, and medroxyprogesterone) prior to and during trial
Excluded: previous use of PTH or sodium fluoride, growth hormone, glucocorticoids or strontium; women with >2+ proteinuria, eGFR < 30, or hypo- or hypercalcemia
Interventions: 3 infusions of 5 mg zoledronic acid (ZA) at 0, 12, and 24 months vs. placebo. All women received oral daily calcium/vitamin D.
Outcomes: Primary: new vertebral fractures (stratum 1) and hip fracture (both strata). Secondary: any nonvertebral fracture, any clinical fracture, clinical vertebral fracture, bone mineral density, markers of bone turnover
Sample size: 7765; 90% power to detect a 50% reduction in vertebral fractures
Randomization: Random permuted blocks within strata
Blinding: Double-blinded

Statistical methods: As treated analysis; Kaplan-Meier, ANCOVA, Fisher's exact test

Results
Participant flow: 7765 randomized (3889 ZA arm, 3876 placebo arm); 3248 ZA group completed follow-up, 3269 placebo group (reasons for not completing follow-up included adverse events, withdrawal of consent, loss to follow-up; numbers not provided); 3875 ZA underwent efficacy analysis, 3861 placebo. Follow-up 3yr.
Baseline data: No significant differences; 21% of patients in both arms with ongoing treatment with non-bisphosphonate osteoporosis medications
Outcomes and estimation: Vertebral fracture rates were 10.9% in placebo vs. 3.3% in treatment group (p<0.001, NNT=13). Hip fracture rates were 2.5% in placebo vs 1.4% in treatment group (p=0.002, NNT=91). Decreases in serum markers in bone turnover and bone density by DEXA were seen in the ZA group.
Ancillary analyses: No effect on overall mortality.
Harms: No differences in jaw osteonecrosis. Flu-like symptoms increased in the week after zoledronic acid infusion. Increase in atrial fibrillation in treatment arm (1.3% vs. 0.5%, p<0.001, NNH=125)

Discussion
Conclusion: Annual zoledronic acid infusions are effective in reducing vertebral and hip fractures in high-risk postmenopausal women. There was an increase in atrial fibrillation in treated patients.
Limitations: Intervention studied against placebo rather than against oral bisphosphonate

Funding: Novartis Pharma (manufacturer of zolendronic acid used in the study)

Commentary   *Marc Wein, MD, PhD, Resident in Internal Medicine*
This HORIZON trial established efficacy for annual zoledronic acid infusions in preventing fractures in high-risk women compared to placebo. Subsequent studies by the same trial group showed that this medication, compared with placebo, reduces mortality in patients following hip fracture [NEJM 2007;357:1799]. Although this study's generalizability is limited as it only included women off glucocorticoids, other studies have clearly established a benefit for bisphosphonates in a wide range of patient populations [Cochrane Database Syst Rev. 2000:CD001347]. The unexpected finding of increased rates of atrial fibrillation in the treatment arm remains controversial and the mechanism is unclear. The major criticism of this study is the appropriateness of a placebo control, as all the patients enrolled clearly qualify for bisphosphonate therapy.

OMEPRAZOLE BEFORE ENDOSCOPY IN PATIENTS WITH GASTROINTESTINAL BLEEDING
Lau J, Leung W, Wu J, et al.
New England Journal of Medicine 2007; 356:1631

Summary: Intravenous omeprazole infusion prior to endoscopy decreases the need for endoscopic intervention and expedites the resolution of upper GI bleeding

Introduction: A neutral gastric pH is vital for clot stability over bleeding arteries.

Objective: "Investigate the effect of the preemptive infusion of omeprazole before endoscopy on the need for endoscopic intervention."

Methods
Trial Design: Randomized controlled trial, double-blind, placebo-controlled (Hong Kong)
Participants: Adult patients with upper GI bleed (melena/hematemesis). Excluded: shock, pregnancy, proton pump inhibitor (PPI) allergy, long-term aspirin use
Interventions: 80-mg IV omeprazole + 8mg/h until endoscopic examination vs. placebo infusion
Outcomes: Need for endoscopic therapy. Secondary: active bleeding at EGD, need for urgent endoscopy, emergent surgery, rebleeding, death, length of stay, transfusion
Sample size: 638 (319 to each group) for 90% power to detect 15% reduction in endoscopic treatment with alpha 0.05
Randomization: computer generated
Blinding: Double-blinded
Statistical methods: Fisher's exact test, Kaplan-Meier method

Results
Participant flow: 638 enrolled, 7 excluded for misdiagnosis and subject withdrawal
Baseline Data: no significant differences
Outcomes and estimation: Fewer patients in the omeprazole group (19.1 vs. 28.4%) required endoscopic intervention (p<0.007). Omeprazole reduced length of stay vs. placebo (p<0.005)
Ancillary analyses: Active bleeding in PPI group was less than in placebo group (p<0.01). No differences in rates of surgery, rebleeding, or death
Harms: None identified

Discussion
Conclusion: Omeprazole infusion before endoscopy reduces the need for endoscopic intervention and decreases rates of active bleeding.
Limitations: Excluded long term aspirin patients; low prevalence of variceal bleeding in study population

Funding: Institute of Digestive Disease

Commentary   *Amit Desai, MD, Resident in Internal Medicine*
This paper provides the evidence for using IV PPIs preemptively in patients presenting with suspected UGIB. However, pre-endoscopic PPI infusion has not been shown to affect mortality, rebleeding, or need for surgery in large systematic reviews [Cochrane Syst Rev.2010:CD005415]. The International Consensus guidelines recommends pre-endoscopic IV PPI infusion and to continue infusions post-endoscopy in patients with high-risk stigmata on endoscopy [Ann Intern Med. 2010; 152:101]. The overall benefits of IV bolus versus continuous IV PPI infusion is still unclear.

PROSPECTIVE RANDOMISED STUDY OF THE EFFECTS OF OCTREOTIDE ON REBLEEDING FROM
OESOPHAGEAL VARICES AFTER ENDOSCOPIC LIGATION
Sung J, Chung SC, Yung MY, et al.
Lancet. 1995; 346: 1666

Summary: Octreotide infusion diminishes rebleeding after variceal band ligation.

Introduction: Rebleeding from esophageal varices after endoscopic ligation with banding is common in the setting of variceal hemorrhage.

Objective: "[To] investigat[e] the efficacy of octreotide infusion as an adjunct to endoscopic variceal ligation to prevent early rebleeding from varices."

Methods
Trial Design: Randomized, single center study (China)
Participants: 100 consecutive patients with endoscopically confirmed esophageal varices and active bleeding or signs of recent hemorrhage (e.g.-clot, cherry red spot); Excluded: history of treated esophageal varices, previous shunt surgery, history of hepatocellular carcinoma, other bleeding source
Interventions: Endoscopic variceal ligation vs. variceal ligation + IV octreotide (50ug bolus at endoscopy, followed by 50ug/hr infusion, for 5days); After these initial treatments, both groups received follow-up endoscopy to ensure obliteration of varices.
Outcomes: Primary: rebleeding. Secondary: initial hemostasis, need for balloon tamponade, transfusion requirement, in-hospital, 30day, 1-yr mortality
Sample size: 100 patients; study powered to detect a reduction in rebleeding rate from 35% to 10% with 80% power and an alpha of 0.05
Randomization: Randomization processes not defined
Blinding: Unblinded
Statistical methods: Intention-to treat analysis; Student's t-test or Pearson's X^2/Fischer's exact tests; Mann-Whitney U for transfusion requirements

Results
Participant flow: 100 patients enrolled, 50 randomized to each treatment group; 3 patients in each group excluded for HCC or gastric variceal bleeding; 3 patients in the variceal ligation group and 1 in the combined therapy group lost to follow-up
Baseline data: No significant differences
Outcomes and estimation: Rates of rebleeding were lower in the ligation plus octreotide group than in the ligation only group (9% vs 38%; p=.0007). Initial hemostasis and transfusion requirements were statistically equivalent between the two groups. Balloon tamponade requirements were higher in the ligation only group. A trend toward lower in-hospital and 30-day mortality was seen in the combined therapy group, but was not statistically significant. Study of 1-yr mortality was incomplete at time of publishing
Ancillary analyses: None
Harms: None identified

Discussion
Conclusion: Octreotide infusion significantly reduced recurrent hemorrhage after endoscopic variceal ligation
Limitations: Octreotide is expensive; optimal duration of therapy is unclear

Funding: Sandoz Pharmaceuticals (maker of Sandostatin, a form of octreotide)

Commentary   *John H. Holden, MD, Resident in Internal Medicine*
In their notable study, Sung et al. show that pharmacologic therapy with octreotide, combined with endoscopic therapy (variceal ligation), may dramatically reduce the risk of variceal rebleeding with few, if any, harms. However, despite showing a promising trend, the study was underpowered to show a statistically significant benefit to mortality with octreotide use. Subsequent meta-analyses have shown a reduced incidence of re-bleeding when pharmacologic therapy is used in conjunction with endoscopic therapy, but have failed to show a clear mortality benefit [Hepatology. 2002; 35:609].

A RANDOMIZED TRIAL OF PREDNISOLONE IN PATIENTS WITH SEVERE ALCOHOLIC HEPATITIS

Ramond MJ, Poynard T, Rueff B, et al.
New England Journal of Medicine. 1992; 326: 507

Summary: Twenty-eight days of prednisolone improves survival in patients with severe alcoholic hepatitis, defined by the presence of encephalopathy or a discriminant function greater than 32.

Introduction Alcoholic hepatitis is associated with an up to 65% in-hospital mortality with few well-studied treatment options.

Objective: "Assess the hypothesis that corticosteroid therapy could improve short-term survival in patients with the severe form of alcoholic hepatitis."

Methods
Trial Design: Randomized, double blinded, 2 centers in France
Participants: Patients with biopsy proven alcoholic hepatitis with encephalopathy or a discriminant function (DF) >32, or both. Excluded: GI bleed, bacterial infection, positive hepatitis B surface Ag, positive HIV antibodies
Interventions: 28 days of 40mg prednisolone treatment vs. placebo
Outcomes: 2 and 6 month mortality
Sample size: 65 patients needed to show 50% reduction in mortality with alpha error of 5% and beta error of 10%
Randomization: Computer generated
Blinding: Double blinded not including pharmacists
Statistical methods: Intention to treat analysis; Parametric (t-test and Fisher's exact test) and nonparametric tests (Mann-Whitney test)

Results
Participant flow: 93 patients with alcoholic hepatitis and DF>32, 61 included in study after exclusions for bleeding, infection, HIV, HBV, cancer
Baseline data: No significant differences.
Outcomes and estimation: 16/29 placebo recipients vs. 4/32 prednisolone recipients died at two months (P=0.001).
Ancillary analyses: 6 mos survival was 84 ±6 % in prednisolone group vs. 45±9% (P=0.002). Significant improvement in prothrombin time, bilirubin, albumin, and Cr was seen in the prednisolone group compared to placebo. Survival was higher in patients treated with prednisolone and those without encephalopathy.
Harms: No serious harm

Discussion
Conclusion: In severe alcoholic hepatitis, Prednisolone increases short term survival.
Limitations: Small study size. The delay from admission to randomization was relatively long (15 days on average) due to delay in liver biopsy results. Because long delays may lead to death, the authors recommend starting prednisolone therapy prior to liver biopsy results and discontinuation if diagnosis not confirmed

Funding: None identified

Commentary   *Tian Gao, MD, Resident in Internal Medicine*
There is ongoing controversy regarding steroid use in alcoholic hepatitis. This study found steroids to be beneficial in patients with severe disease, defined as the presence of encephalopathy or a discriminant function>32. In a meta-analysis of 5 RCTs, glucocorticoids did appear to reduce overall mortality, but only in patients with a discriminant function >32. [*Gut.* 2011; 60:225] The 2010 ACG/AASLD guideline recommends the use of glucocorticoids as first line therapy except in patients with renal failure or contraindication to steroids. Therapy should be continued for 21 days. The decision to stop prednisolone due to lack of efficacy can be assessed by calculating the Lille score after 7 days of treatment. Despite its benefit, prednisolone can be ineffective in approximately 40% of patients with alcoholic hepatitis. Pentoxifylline, an anti-TNF agent and potential alternative treatment for those patients with a contraindication to steroids, has mixed results in alcoholic hepatitis and in a recent small trial did not improve 6-month survival when added to prednisolone [*JAMA.* 2013; 310: 1033]. In a separate trial, addition of *N*-acetylcysteine to prednisolone also did not improve 6-month survival compared to prednisolone alone [*NEJM*; 2011; 365:1781]

INTRAVENEOUS N-ACETYLCYSTEINE IMPROVES TRANSPLANT-FREE SURVIVAL IN EARLY STAGE NON-ACETAMINOPHEN ACUTE LIVER FAILURE
Lee W, Hynan L, Rossaro L, et al.
Gastroenterology 2009; 137:856

Summary: Intravenous N-Acetylcysteine increases transplant-free survival in non-acetaminophen-associated acute liver failure with low grade encephalopathy.

Introduction: Intravenous N-Acetylcysteine (IV NAC) can prevent liver damage in acetaminophen induced acute liver failure (ALF) when given within 24 hours.

Objective: "Treatment with NAC may benefit patients with non-acetaminophen related acute liver failure. Our research hypothesis was that patients receiving NAC would have higher overall survival rates then those receiving placebo."

Methods
Trial Design: Prospective, randomized, double-blinded, placebo-controlled, multicenter (US)
Participants: Adult patients with ALF as defined by evidence of encephalopathy and coagulopathy (INR > 1.5) for < 24 weeks. Excluded: 1) known or suspected acetaminophen overdose 2) previous NAC use 3) shock liver 4) liver failure related to pregnancy 5) refractory hypotension 6) septic shock 7) imminent liver transplant (in <8 hours)
Interventions: IV NAC + 5% Dextrose (150mg/kg/h x 1 hr + 12.5mg/kg/h x 4 hrs + 6.25 mg/kg/h x 67 hrs) vs. 5% dextrose alone
Outcomes: Overall survival at 3 weeks after randomization. Secondary: tansplant free survival and transplant rate.
Sample size: 170 (to achieve 80% power with alpha= 0.05)
Randomization: Stratified by coma categories (I-II vs III-IV) and then randomized by site
Statistical methods: Intention to treat analysis: chi-square and Student t-test (1-sided for overall survival and transplant free survival, otherwise 2 sided), odds ratio, log-rank test

Results
Participant flow: 820 eligible, 558 were initially excluded, 89 were later excluded for various reasons. 173 patients were randomized and completed the study, 92 to placebo and 81 to NAC: this group difference was due to randomization by coma grade and site.
Baseline data: No significant differences based on etiology of ALF. Placebo group had more females and longer median time between jaundice and encephalopathy (12 vs. 7 days)
Outcomes and estimation: Overall survival at 3 weeks was 70% for NAC and 66% for placebo (p=.283). Transplant-free survival was 40% in NAC group and 27% in placebo (p=.043). Only 63% of patients in the placebo arm and 59% in the NAC arm completed 72 hours of therapy.
Ancillary analyses: Transplant free survival broken down by coma grade: Grade I-II: 52% in NAC group vs 30% in placebo (p=.01). Grade III-IV: 9% in NAC group vs 22% in placebo (p=.912). By etiology, drug induced liver injury and HBV showed improved survival outcomes compared to autoimmune or indeterminate causes.
Harms: 1 patient in each treatment group experienced bronchospasm

Discussion
Conclusion: Improved transplant-free survival at 3 weeks and at 1 year was observed with the use of NAC for the treatment of non-acetaminophen related ALF. The benefit was confined to those with low grade (grade I-II) encephalopathy.
Limitations: none identified

Funding: National Institute of Diabetes and Digestive and Kidney Diseases

---

Commentary   *Jessica Ravikoff, MD, Resident in Internal Medicine*
This paper presents the only data on the use of NAC in non-acetaminophen related ALF. While transplant remains the mainstay of therapy, this article has provided physicians with an additional therapeutic option. The benefit of NAC in this study was restricted to those with low-grade encephalopathy, suggesting the intractability of higher grade encephalopathy and the need for transplantation. The study was well designed; however, of 820 eligible patients, over 600 were excluded. Although data on the etiology of ALF was collected, the low numbers of each etiology precluded subgroup analysis. NAC has been studied in vivo and in vitro and has been shown to be relatively safe. Larger studies are needed to determine if specific etiologies of non-acetaminophen related ALF are more responsive to treatment with IV NAC.

EFFECT OF INTRAVENOUS ALBUMIN ON RENAL IMPAIRMENT AND MORTALITY IN PATIENTS WITH
CIRRHOSIS AND SPONTANEOUS BACTERIAL PERITONITIS
Sort P, Navasa M, Arroyo V, et al.
New England Journal of Medicine. 1999; 341: 403

Summary: Intravenous albumin on day 1 and day 3 improves mortality in a select population of cirrhotics with spontaneous bacterial peritonitis.

Introduction: Renal failure due to decreased effective arterial blood volume is common in patients with cirrhosis and spontaneous bacterial peritonitis (SBP).

Objective: "To determine whether plasma volume expansion with intravenous albumin prevents renal impairment and reduces mortality in these patients."

Methods
Trial Design: Randomized, multicenter (Spain)
Participants: Adults with cirrhosis and ascites neutrophil count > 250. Excluded: antibiotic treatment within one week, shock, GI bleed, grade 3-4 encephalopathy, cardiac failure, HIV infection, other causes of nephropathy, serum creatinine > 3 mg/dl
Interventions: IV cefotaxime vs. IV cefotaxime + IV albumin (1.5g/kg on day 1 and 1.0g/kg on day 3)
Outcomes: Primary: nonreversible deterioration of renal function defined as >50% increase in BUN or Cr. Secondary: mortality
Sample size: 100; powered to detect the development of renal impairment
Randomization: Concealed from investigators; independent random number generation at each center
Blinding: Unblinded
Statistical methods: Intention-to-treat analysis; chi-square test or Student's t-test

Results
Participant flow: 199 enrolled, 73 excluded prior to randomization; the remaining 126 were randomized and completed the protocol
Baseline data: no significant differences
Outcomes and estimation: Renal impairment developed in 33% controls vs. 10% in the intervention arm (p = 0.0002). 29% in control group died vs. 10% in intervention prior to discharge (p = 0.01), a significant trend which was also seen at three months.
Ancillary analyses: 78% of patients who developed renal impairment died during hospitalization; plasma renin activity was higher in control arm; arterial blood pressure did not significantly change after albumin infusion.
Harms: None identified

Discussion
Conclusion: Intravenous albumin in addition to antibiotics to treat SBP in cirrhotics diminishes the incidence of renal impairment and mortality.
Limitations: Albumin is expensive and optimal dosing is unknown.

Funding: Fondo de Investigacion Sanitaria, Spain

Commentary *Jonathan Soverow, MD, MPH, Resident in Internal Medicine*
Over a decade old, this paper still dictates treatment of SBP and represents one of the few data-driven uses of albumin, an expensive blood product whose use is controversial in the critically ill. The study is well-designed and internally valid, combining standard antibiotics with large doses of albumin, which appear to reduce mortality by preventing renal failure without affecting systemic blood pressure. However, the inclusion/exclusion criteria make practical use of this study challenging. "Cirrhosis" is not defined, and the broad exclusion criteria eliminated 40% of the initial patients with "cirrhosis" and SBP. Despite this, no further studies updating optimal dosing of intravenous albumin in the setting of SBP have been done [NEJM 2009; 361: 1279]; a meta-analysis of 4 RCTs using albumin affirms the mortality benefit seen in this trial as well as a reduction in renal failure. [*Clin Gastroenterol Hepatol.* 2013; 11:123.]

RIFAXIMIN TREATMENT IN HEPATIC ENCEPHALOPATHY
Bass NM, Mullen KD, Sanyal A, et al.
New England Journal of Medicine. 2010; 362: 1071

Summary: In cirrhotic patients with recurrent hepatic encephalopathy, rifaximin added to lactulose reduces recurrence and the risk of hospitalization for encephalopathy compared with lactulose alone.

<u>Introduction:</u> Rifaximin is effective in the treatment of hepatic encephalopathy (HE), but its role in secondary prevention of HE is uncertain

Objective: "[To evaluate] the efficacy and safety of rifaximin, used concomitantly with lactulose, for the maintenance of remission from episodes of hepatic encephalopathy in outpatients with a recent history of recurrent, overt hepatic encephalopathy."

Methods
Trial Design: Multicenter (US, Canada, Russia), randomized, double-blind, placebo-controlled phase 3 trial.
Participants: Adults with $\geq$ 2 episodes of HE in the last 6 months, now in remission from HE, and MELD $\leq$ 25. Excluded: expected liver transplant within 1 month, presence of gastrointestinal hemorrhage or TIPS in last 3 months, chronic renal insufficiency (Cr>2 mg/dl), respiratory insufficiency, anemia (Hgb <8 g/dl), electrolyte abnormality (Na<125 mmol/L, Ca>10 mg/dl, K<2.5 mmol/L), intercurrent infection
Interventions: Rifaximin 550 mg BID + lactulose or placebo + lactulose for 6 months.
Outcomes: Time to first breakthrough episode of HE measured by Conn Score and standardized asterixis grade. Secondary: time to first hospitalization involving HE.
Sample size: 299; powered to show superiority of rifaximin over placebo.
Randomization: Concealed from investigators; randomized at 70 investigative sites
Statistical methods: Intention-to-treat analysis; Cox proportional-hazards model; Kaplan-Meier

Results
Participant flow: 299 patients randomized; all were included in intention-to-treat populations
Baseline data: Rifaximin group 53.6% male v. placebo group 67.3%. Majority: white, <65 years, MELD 11-18. ~91% lactulose use in both groups.
Outcomes and estimation: Rifaximin reduced the risk of a breakthrough HE event compared to placebo (22.1% v. 45.9%; HR 0.42; p<0.001) and reduced hospitalization involving HE (13.6% v. 22.6%; HR 0.50; p=0.01)
Ancillary analyses: Consistent results across all subgroups.
Harms: Adverse events not significantly different between rifaximin and placebo groups. *C. difficile* infection in 2 rifaximin patients (with existing risk factors), zero placebo patients.

Discussion
Conclusion: Rifaximin protects against recurrent hepatic encephalopathy and reduces the risk of encephalopathy-related hospitalizations.
Limitations: Authors do not comment.

Funding: Salix Pharmaceuticals (makers of Xifaxin, a branded version of rifaximin)

Commentary   *Zachary A. Zator, MD, Resident in Internal Medicine*
Before this article, rifaximin had only been evaluated as a treatment for acute HE. This study was the first to show that it is also efficacious in the prevention of recurrent HE. However, the study criteria, which eliminate patients with CKD, anemia, and established HE precipitants such as recent GI bleeds and infection, make full generalizability difficult. On the other hand, the study does define a specific population for whom prophylaxis with both rifaximin and lactulose can prevent recurrent HE. It does not assess rifaximin monotherapy or HE due to acute liver failure. Since ~90% of patients were taking lactulose prior to study enrollment, this trial supports the use of rifaximin in addition to lactulose for the prevention of HE in cirrhotics with stable disease and MELD scores <25 who are not awaiting transplant. Although rifaximin is more costly than lactulose, the reduction in hospitalization involving HE may ultimately make it cost effective. Future cost-benefit analyses are therefore warranted.

NORFLOXACIN PREVENTS BACTERIAL INFECTION IN CIRRHOTICS WITH GASTROINTESINAL HEMORRHAGE

Soriano G, Guarner C, Tomas A, et al.
Gastroenterology. 1992;103:1267

Summary: Prophylaxis with norfloxacin in cirrhotic patients with gastrointestinal hemorrhage reduces the incidence of bacterial infections.

Introduction: Bacterial infections, typically with enteric aerobic gram negative organisms, are a frequent cause of morbidity and mortality among cirrhotic patients. Gastrointestinal hemorrhage increases this risk.

Objective: "To assess the efficacy of selective intestinal decontamination with norfloxacin in the prevention of bacterial infections in cirrhotic patients with gastrointestinal hemorrhage."

Methods
Trial Design: Randomized, prospective, single center (Spain)
Participants: Adults with cirrhosis admitted for gastrointestinal hemorrhage. Excluded: patients with signs of infection on admission, antibiotic exposure in the previous 2 weeks, outside hospital transfers
Interventions: Norfloxacin 400mg BID po x 7 days with repeat course if re-bleeding. Antibiotics were started after endoscopy
Outcomes: Incidence of bacterial infections during hospitalization; mortality
Sample size: 119 included in analysis; power calculation not reported
Randomization: Not reported
Blinding: Unblinded
Statistical methods: As-treated analysis; Student's t or chi-square test; patients who died or had surgery within 24 hours were not analyzed

Results
Participant flow: 128 randomized, 8 patients excluded because of death or surgery within 24hrs, 1 patient excluded because he left hospital AMA within 8 hrs of admission; 119 (60 treatment group, 59 control) were analyzed.
Baseline data: No significant differences; majority of bleeding from esophageal varices
Outcomes and estimation: Six infections developed in 6 patients in treatment group vs. 26 infections in 22 patients in control group (10% vs. 37.2%, p=0.001). The majority of infections were spontaneous bacterial perotinitis, bacteremia or urinary tract infections. Mortality in treatment group was 6.6% vs. 11.8% in controls (non-significant).
Ancillary analyses: Norfloxacin reduced the incidence of bacteremia (0% vs 10%) and urinary tract infection (0% vs 18.6%) compared to no antibiotic prophylaxis. There was no significant difference in the incidence of spontaneous bacterial peritonitis, pneumonia, or possible infections.
Harms: None identified.

Discussion
Conclusion: Prophylaxis with norfloxacin in cirrhotic patients with gastrointestinal hemorrhage decreased the incidence of infection and should be considered for all cirrhotic patients with GI bleeding.
Limitations: Small sample size limited the ability to detect differences in mortality.

Funding: Not disclosed

<u>*Commentary*</u>   *Michelle Long, MD, Resident in Internal Medicine*
Written in the early 90s, this paper represents the first RCT demonstrating the efficacy of antibiotics for prophylaxis of infection in cirrhotic patients with gastrointestinal hemorrhage. Subsequent studies have shown the benefit of other antibiotics for the prophylaxis of bacterial infections in cirrhotics with gastrointestinal hemorrhage, including ciprofloxacin, ofloxacin, amoxicillin/clavulanic acid, cefotaxime, and ceftriaxone. Further studies have also documented a reduction in recurrent gastrointestinal bleeding in patients treated with antibiotics. It should also be noted that in this study, the protection from infection seen with norfloxacin was likely due to reduction in nosocomial infections. Recently, the epidemiology of bacterial infections in cirrhotic patients has changed with an increase in infections from gram positive cocci and gram negative bacteria resistant to quinolone therapy. [Gastroenterology. 2006; 131: 1049]